S0-ARM-362

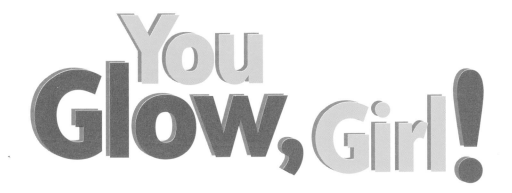

You Glow, Girl!

The Ultimate Health & Skin Care Guide for Teens

Dianne York-Goldman
and Mitchel P. Goldman, M.D.

Quality Medical Publishing, Inc.

ST. LOUIS, MISSOURI 2000

You Glow Girl! Web site address:
www.youglowgirl.com

Copyright © 2000 by York-Goldman Enterprises, Inc.

All rights reserved. Reproduction of the material herein in any form requires the written permission of the publisher.

PUBLISHER   Karen Berger
EDITOR   Beth Campbell
MANUSCRIPT EDITOR   George Mary Gardner
ASSISTANT EDITOR   Kristen Volkmann
TEXT & COVER DESIGN   Articulate Graphics
PHOTOGRAPHY   Noel Grady

Quality Medical Publishing, Inc.
11970 Borman Drive, Suite 222
St. Louis, Missouri 63146
Tel: 800-423-6865
Web site: www.qmp.com

LIBRARY OF CONGRESS CATALOGING-IN-PUBLICATION DATA

Pending

ISBN 1-57626-094-1

AG/W/W

5   4   3   2   1

For our daughters, Risa and Melissa,
and all their friends.

A portion of the profits from this book
go to children's charities.

Here's what people are saying about *You Glow, Girl!*

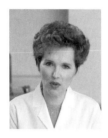

This book should be required reading for every teen seeking advice on the care of their skin.

Helen M. Torok, M.D.
HMT Dermatology Associates, Inc.
Medina, Ohio

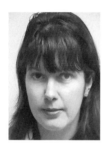

You Glow, Girl! is based on the Goldmans' combined, extensive experience in the world of beauty, physical fitness . . . and derma-tology. They write in a way that is easily understood . . . and convey a great deal of important information succinctly and personally. Their attention to teens' concerns with self-esteem is refreshing. This is an excellent resource for both teenagers and women who care about them.

Margaret Weiss, M.D.
Dermatology Associates of Baltimore
Baltimore, Maryland

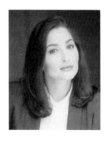

I only wish that I could have read this book when I was a teenager. My generation was clueless. I could have saved myself from adoles-cent rituals involving slathering my skin with baby oil and dousing my hair in lemon juice before sun bathing—not to mention all the pimples operated on with straight pins.

Reneé McNeil
Senior Airline Flight Attendant and Model

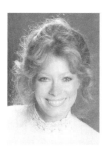

I don't know of anyone more qualified to write a book geared to teens than the Goldmans.

Nancy Burkett
President, Burkett Talent Agency, Inc.
Mission Viejo, California

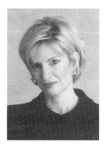

If young women (and men) would practice the skin tips outlined in the Goldmans' book, the use of dermatologic laser surgery to reverse the marks of aging and acne would become obsolete. Don't let the ravages of excessive sun exposure and poor skin management cause you to become a victim of wrinkled, sun-spotted, and acne-scarred skin. This guide is just the place to start when planning, implementing, and maintaining a proper skin care routine.

Tina S. Alster, M.D.
Dermatologist and Laser Surgeon
Author of *The Essential Guide to Cosmetic Laser Surgery*
Washington, D.C.

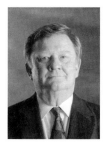

I would challenge you to read this . . . compelling book, and incorporate the Goldmans' advice into your life-style.

John M. Yarborough, Jr., M.D.
Dermatologist
New Orleans, Louisiana

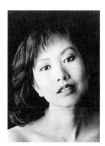

When it comes to being . . . and staying beautiful, Dianne York-Goldman wrote the book—literally!

Lucy Lin
Actress
Manhattan Beach, California

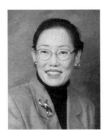

This is the era of self-help. Teenagers want to know what they can do for themselves. However, it is so confusing when one tries to choose the best products. The Goldmans make it easy to understand the nature of skin, hair, and nails and consequently make it easier to choose the right products. Anyone . . . will love reading this book.

Lenore S. Kakita, M.D.
Dermatologist
Glendale, California

Being healthy and feeling attractive contributes to self-confidence . . . this is what the Goldmans' book is about. . . . Readers are provided with tips and helpful advice to advance their sense of style and improve upon their own beauty.

Bettie B. Youngs, Ph.D.
Author of *How to Develop Self-Esteem in Your Child* and *Taste Berry Tales*
Del Mar, California

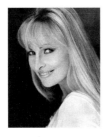

You Glow, Girl! *is a book every teen needs to own.*

Melanie Good
Actress and Model

The Goldmans' advice to young women teaches them important health and beauty tips that will promote confidence for the rest of their lives.

Allee Newhoff
Senior Agent
Irene Marie Model Agency
Miami, Florida and New York, New York

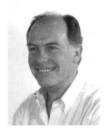

You Glow, Girl! *is an excellent source of medically accurate information written in an understandable and entertaining style.*

Leonardo Corcos, M.D.
Adjunct Professor
University of Sassari
Florence, Italy

Preface

The idea for this book began innocently enough: We thought it would not only fill a crying need, but also be loads of fun to write a skin care guide specifically for teenage women. Certainly, neither of us had seen anything on the subject that was completely suited to the teens we knew, even though it's a snap to find any number of admirable volumes on similar topics for *older women*. The reason for this, of course, is basic supply and demand. Mature women, you see, want what their teenage daughters (and nieces and granddaughters) enjoy now: younger looking skin. *And they want it bad!* Writers and publishers, for their part, know a good audience when they see one, and have responded with books enough to stock the shelves of a small local library.

Now, we'd love to tell you that older women read more about skin care because they've grown wiser with the passing years. But all too often, we suspect, their interest has been aroused not by any positive impulse but by one or more of the troubling signs that result from damaged or aging skin—lines at the corners of the eyes and mouth that seem to deepen every day, a scaliness on the back of the hands that no lotion or cream can smooth, a persistently sallow, pasty complexion, or, worst of all, the sudden appearance of blotchy red patches signaling the early stages of skin cancer.

The great majority of skin problems, in fact, don't start becoming outwardly noticeable until we hit our early to mid-30s. Prior to that, the skin exhibits an almost miraculous capacity to bounce back from the hardships imposed on it by our poor eating habits, overexposure to the elements, lack of proper rest, and haphazard skin care. Compare, for example, the two or three days needed for a 16-year-old's skin to recover from a mild case of sunburn to the week or more that might be required to heal the skin of her 40-year-old mother. Or take the same two women and look at them side by side the morning following a bad night's sleep. Whose complexion is fresher and clearer, say, an hour or so after waking? The 16-year-old's, in nine cases out of ten, because young skin is generally more supple, more vibrant, and more forgiving than skin that's been around the block a few times.

The resilience of young skin, however, can be dangerously misleading, since so many common skin conditions take years—and sometimes even decades—to become apparent. So while it may seem, at first glance, that teens simply don't have as much need for skin care advice as older women, quite the opposite is actually true. Teens who treat their youth as a kind of "summer vacation" from skin care are setting themselves up for problems that will likely surface in early adulthood and worsen as they age. In the long run, then, it's far healthier, far easier, and far less expensive to preserve the youthful skin you possess now than to correct flawed skin in your 30s, 40s, 50s and beyond.

Consequently, our primary goal in this book is to help teens develop skin-care habits—and to a lesser extent life-style habits—that will not only enable them to look their best today but also to retain their youthful good looks for a lifetime. To that end, we've pooled our expertise in dermatology, modeling, and acting to present both sides of the "health" and "beauty" story in the pages that follow. Along the way, we've tried to strike a reasonable balance between providing sound, scientifically responsible information, on the one hand, and allowing ourselves (and, hopefully, you!) to have some fun on the other. After all, one of the most charming aspects of beauty—and its relentless pursuit by women of all ages—is that it combines our most serious and frivolous sides in nearly equal measure!

The first part of the book covers the basics of skin care. Here, you'll learn how the skin works, how to cleanse it for best results, how to protect it from sun damage, and how to deal intelligently with acne and related skin problems. From there, you'll venture to the outer limits of the skin as we cover the essentials of both hair care and nail care, including a thorough examination of common problems that afflict these regions. We'll show how to spot trouble early on, deal with it correctly, and, best of all, prevent it from recurring in the future. Finally, the book's third and last section caps things off by addressing diet, exercise, stress, and rest, as well as the critically important, but often overlooked, question of how to choose the right dermatologist for you.

Now that you've had a sneak preview of what's to come, it's time to *get glowing!* Our only hope is that you gain as many insights and derive as much enjoyment from your reading as we did from our research and writing.

Dianne York-Goldman
Mitchel P. Goldman, M.D.

Acknowledgments

As with any book, many people in addition to the authors are responsible for its final form. As much as we would like to, it is impossible for us to acknowledge every person who has given us ideas or provided information. We sincerely apologize for any omissions.

Mark Blethroad spent countless hours providing research, ideas, and his invaluable writing talent for this project. He transformed the early pages into a text that teenagers as well as adults will find interesting and easy to read. Although the father of a young son, he somehow knew how to speak the language of our teenaged daughters. We also give many thanks to his wife and partner, Beth Campbell, our editor. Beth's guidance, patience, and unwavering diligence in completing this project went above and beyond the call of duty.

A picture *is* worth a thousand words, and no one does it better than Noel Grady, our personal friend and photographer. Noel's decades of experience photographing young women and models truly made the book come alive. Thanks also to Diana Stewart for providing the candid, real-life photos that give this book so much fun and flair. Also, Joel and Sharon Harris of *Articulate Graphics* were superb in their creation of the style and design implementation.

Technical and research support was provided by Diane Foster of *Neutrogena*; Jeff Nugent, Eileen Higgens, and Donna Shapiro of *Revlon/Almay*; Bill Humphries and Doug Abel of *Allergan*; Jonah Shacknai, Rick Havens, and Ralph Bohrer of *Medicis*; Mary Madden of *Galderma*; Robert Bitterman, Keith Greathouse, and Elaine Ward of *Dermik*; and Drs. Richard Fitzpatrick and Kimberly Butterwick of *SkinMedica*.

Our good friend, Tony Ray, hairstylist to the stars and owner of *Stainless* of Rancho Santa Fe, California, freely shared his experience and hair pearls with us. Many other close friends, including Dr. Bettie Youngs, Maria Camille, Darlene Dise-Brucker, Peter Greenberg, Rudy Maxa, Judith Bardwick, Nadine Tosk, Carol Clark, and Lynn McMahan, provided the advice and encouragement needed to help us persevere.

Finally, we owe our gratitude to all the teenaged patients and proteges who have touched our lives over the years. It is our hope that this book can give back to them some of the joy we have experienced from the knowledge that we were able to play a small part in their maturation.

Contents

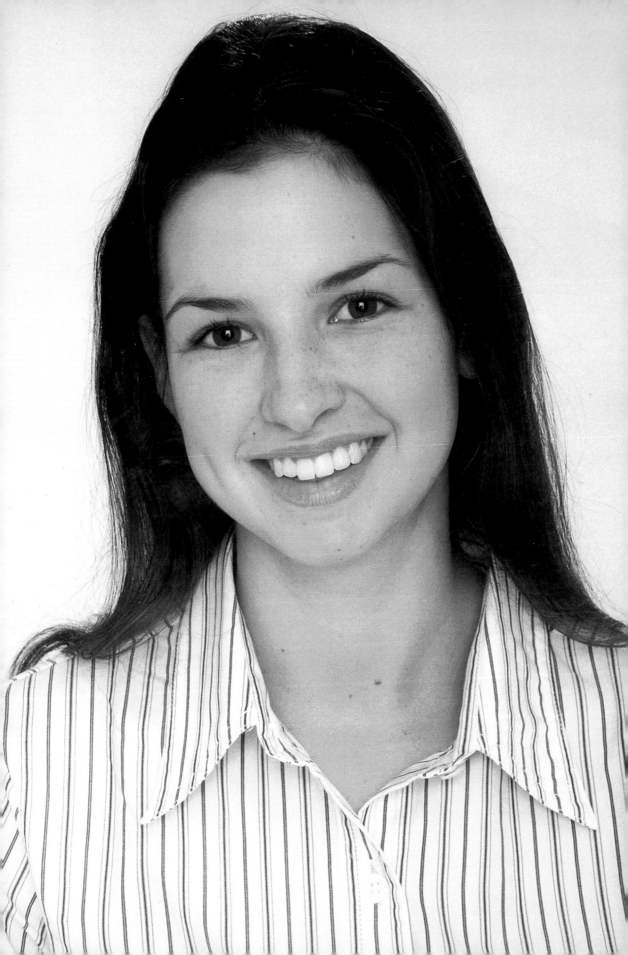

Skin 101: The Basics

These days, the subject of skin is definitely *in*. If you doubt it, just surf the channels on your cable TV or scan the pages of nearly any popular magazine. Our guess is that you'll catch everything from glossy cosmetics ads and dire skin cancer warnings to intricately tattooed torsos and piercings in places no woman has dared to pierce before. Here in America, especially, it seems obvious that we're showing more skin, decorating it more elaborately, and—in some extreme cases—stretching it to the absolute limit for the purposes of beauty and self-expression.

Now, on a certain level, none of this should come as too huge a shock to anyone. After all, people throughout history and across cultures have always preoccupied themselves with the appearance of their skin. We understand almost intuitively that what others see first is neither our warm heart nor our razor-sharp mind but our skin. Skin is a badge we wear day in and day out: It delivers tell-tale messages about our overall health, acts as a pipeline for all of our senses, protects us against the elements, and influences profoundly not only how others perceive us but also how we perceive ourselves. To that extent, our timeless fascination with skin (and skin care!) is both natural and healthy.

This book tells you how to achieve *great-looking* skin. Despite the old saying that "beauty is only skin deep," we assume that most people would like to look great—or, at a minimum, better than they did the day before. So we've combined the medical expertise and technical knowledge of a leading dermatologist (Mitch) with the aesthetic sense and beauty savvy of a professional model and actress (Dianne) to put you on the path to skin nirvana.

Below:

Women have been enhancing their beauty for centuries.

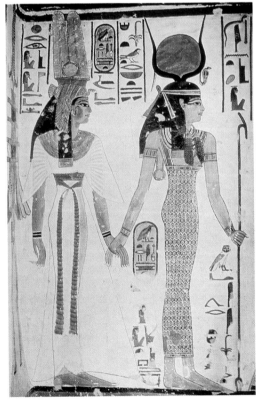

Some of the ideas we'll share with you have been around for ages. Others are the product of the most recent scientific research. Some of the topics we'll cover are chiefly medical in nature. Others deal with strictly cosmetic issues. But no matter what the content of a specific section or chapter, our objective throughout is to present the kind of balanced, in-depth advice that will help you enjoy beautiful skin now, and for years to come. Step one in that process is to learn more about how our skin is constructed and how it functions in the human body.

AN OVERVIEW OF THE SKIN

Among the most commonly asked "trick" questions used on television game shows and in biology pop quizzes is this little gem: What is the largest organ of the human body? The answer, as you might have guessed, is the skin. The question often stumps people because when we think of bodily organs we tend to picture the dramatic action of, say, the heart pumping blood or the lungs processing oxygen. The skin, in comparison, appears to be nothing more than a protective wrapper for all the important work being done by the "real" organs inside.

Of course, it's true that protection of internal organs is a key function of the skin. But this passive view of how it works couldn't be farther removed from reality. Just like other major bodily organs, our skin operates nonstop in an active, dynamic fashion. It helps keep us properly hydrated by regulating retention of salt and water through the sweat glands. It assists in flushing impurities from our system through the action of the blood vessels, oil glands, sweat glands, and pores. It constantly renews itself by sloughing off dead cells and manufacturing new ones. It filters the sun's UV light rays so we don't get cooked like a burger on the grill. It reacts and adjusts to changes in temperature and humidity, acting as a thermostat for the body to cool us down when it's hot and warm us up when it's not. It . . . Well, we could go on and on about all the crucial tasks the skin performs—and we will discuss some of them in more detail later—but we think you probably have the big picture for now: The skin is one busy organ, despite what outward appearances seem to suggest!

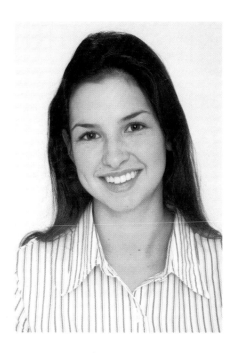

Above:
She's got "the glow!"

THE LAYERS OF THE SKIN

The skin has three principal layers[1] each with a name more imposing than the last: subcutaneous, dermis, epidermis. (Couldn't they have gone with, oh, *bottom*, *middle*, and *top*? Naw, too easy; everyone would remember those!) But tongue-twisting terms notwithstanding, let's examine each layer, one by one, to gain a fuller understanding of how the entire apparatus goes about its business. Once we've done that, we'll have a sound basis for making smarter, better informed skin care decisions across the board.

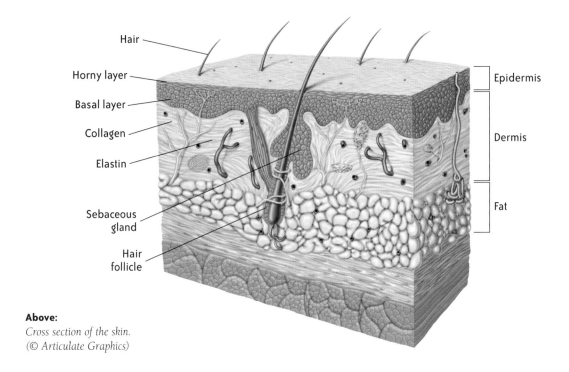

Hair

Horny layer

Basal layer

Collagen

Elastin

Sebaceous
gland

Hair
follicle

Epidermis

Dermis

Fat

Above:
Cross section of the skin.
(© Articulate Graphics)

Since so many of the skin's most vital chores happen below the surface, it's instructive to take a bottoms-up look at its construction. The analogy we like to make, though it's admittedly imperfect, is to compare the skin to a carpet.

At the bottom, or base, of the carpet lies the padding, which provides cushioning and insulation to the layers immediately above and below. In the skin, we refer to this padding as the *subcutaneous* layer, which is simply a specialized way of saying that it lies under the *dermis* (or middle layer, which we will deal with shortly). The subcutaneous layer is composed primarily of fat, and its main mission in life is to protect our tender internal organs by dampening the effect of both external shocks— someone, heaven forbid, slaps you, or you fall on your butt rollerblading—and exposure to the cold. Ask any frostbite victim, and our bet is that they'll tell you a tad too much subcutaneous fat is preferable to not enough, which should be food for thought the next time you want to diet down to a smaller dress size!

The middle and thickest layer of the skin, the *dermis*, roughly corresponds to the backing on a carpet. Like carpet backing—and like other types of connective tissue in the body—the dermis is composed of very durable, resilient, fibrous material, and its principal function is to provide shape and support to the outermost layer everyone else sees, much in the manner that the bones provide a framework for our muscles. Significantly, this layer also houses our sweat and oil glands, the skin's blood vessels, hair roots, and more nerve endings than you could count in a lifetime (which is why you get "goose flesh" when you're chilly or when the right person smiles at you). Without the dermis, the skin could not receive vital nutrients and oxygen or dispose of poisonous waste products.

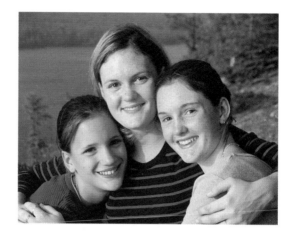

Because of its structural and vascular (or blood-supplying) functions, the overall vitality of the dermis greatly impacts the outward appearance of our skin's surface. Two of its more noteworthy components in this regard, which you may have read or heard about before, are *collagen* and *elastin*. Both are fibrous proteins, and each plays an essential role in skin health. Collagen fibers keep the skin firm, while elastin fibers, as the name implies, keep skin tight by giving it the capacity to spring back into shape when we "pinch an inch." If your skin completely lacked these crucial fibers, do you know what would happen if someone poked a finger into your stomach? The indent made by their fingertip would stay there until you physically pulled the skin back out. Bizarre, but true!

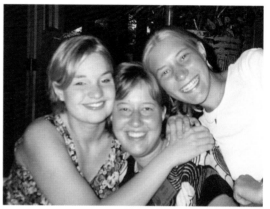

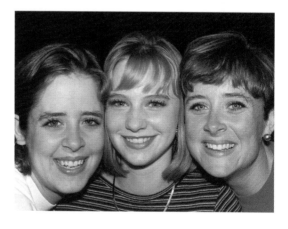

In real life, something not too awfully different from this example occurs. As we age, and more important, as our skin is exposed to sunlight, our collagen and elastin fibers loosen and ultimately are destroyed. The result: wrinkles. Look at any of the older women around you—your mother, your grandmoth-

Above:
Take a look at your parents and grandparents to get an idea of how you will age. Genetics are important, but read on for tips on how to slow the aging process.

ers, aunts, teachers, whomever— and you will see that they have wrinkles to one degree or another. And, if you check with them, we have few doubts that the ones with the most wrinkles are those who got the most sun and spent the most time outdoors when they were YOUR AGE. So while you may have no wrinkles today, you'll need to make the right lifestyle choices and take appropriate protective measures now to prevent them from developing in the future.

We intend to show you ways to preserve your smooth, tight, wrinkle-free skin throughout this book, but especially in the chapter on tanning, which is must reading for all young women who enjoy water sports, laying out, or just being in the great outdoors. For the present, however, let's move on to the final and outermost layer of the skin.

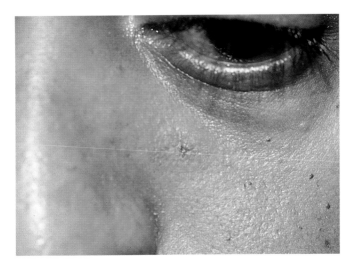

Above:
Some rashes may go away on their own. Those that linger for more than a few days should be treated by a dermatologist.

At last, we've reached the carpet's surface, the part we want to be as smooth, unblemished and aesthetically appealing as possible—the *epidermis*. Special skin cells called *keratinocytes* make up most of this layer, which varies greatly in thickness depending on the particular area of the body in question. In the eyelids, for instance, the epidermis is only about as thick as a sheet of ordinary writing paper. But in the soles of our feet it widens to the approximate thickness of the leather used in a wallet or a purse.

Skin thickness is an important factor to consider when we do scads of everyday things like washing, moisturizing, using makeup, and applying sunscreen. The skin around our eyes, for example, is extremely thin and therefore very sensitive to chemicals. So common sense dictates that we use only the gentlest soaps and purest moisturizers there. Conversely, the layer of epidermis covering our hands, feet, and back is fairly thick and tough. Here it's OK—and even preferable—to take advantage of the greater cleansing power and hydrating action offered,

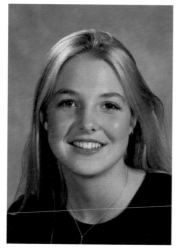
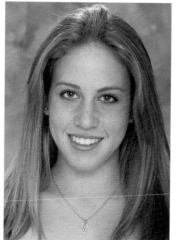
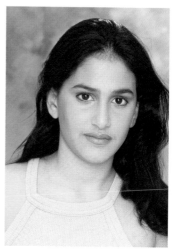

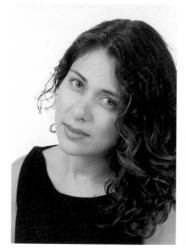
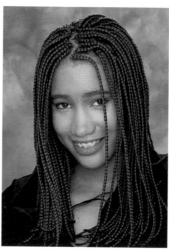

Above and left:
Melanocytes, or pigment cells, determine skin tone.

respectively, by stronger soaps and thicker moisturizers. How do we know when we've applied the wrong product to a specific area of the skin? Simple: Our epidermis tells us so by developing a red, scaly rash like the one illustrated on the facing page. When you see this kind of rash, check your toiletries and try to identify the offending item or items. Then substitute with something gentler.

Besides the keratinocytes noted earlier, the epidermis also contains *melanocytes*, more commonly known as pigment cells. These generate *melanin*, a brownish, black pigment contained in the tissue of many animals, including us humans. When melanocytes are stimulated by sunlight or by our body's own hormones, they swing into action, producing melanin and pumping it up to cells near the skin's surface through tentacle-like appendages called *dendrites*. Generally speaking, the more melanocytes we possess and the more densely melanin is packed within our pigment cells, the darker our skin, hair, and eye color will tend to be. Also, certain types of melanocytes are notably more active than others, which likewise contributes to a relatively darker complexion in people who have them. Since melanin *partially* filters and thereby lessens the damage caused by UV light, a person's capacity to produce it will, to a great degree, determine his or her ability to safely withstand the sun's harmful rays. This explains why darker skinned people are typically less susceptible, though certainly not immune, to sunburn than lighter skinned folks are.

Individual variation in the number, type, and capacity of our melanocytes, then, accounts for the fact that while human skin comes in a few basic colors (pale, tan, yellow, brown, etc.), it exhibits an astounding range of hues and shades within each group—so many, in fact, that even the most gifted painter would have a hard time reproducing a fraction of them precisely. Our attitude is that any color is great; the key is for the color to be uniform. Blotchy color indicates that the pigment cells we've been talking about are either irritated or damaged, a subject we'll cover at greater length when we discuss sun damage and other skin problems.

Finally, it's worth noting that some types of spots, such as freckles, birthmarks, and most moles, are perfectly natural in healthy skin. If you wish to cover them up or make them appear more even, a few well-placed dabs of concealer will

Below:

Freckles and moles are normal. You can play up these features for a unique or striking beauty look (think Nicole Kidman or Cindy Crawford), or you may wish to disguise them.

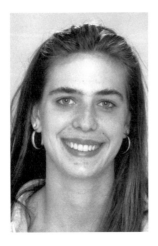

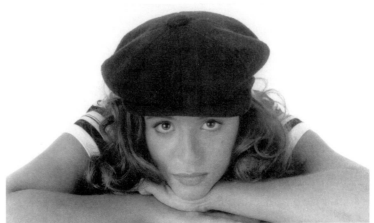

usually do the trick. But if not, that's fine too; after all, Cindy Crawford seems to cope quite well with her mole, and we've all known a cute guy or two with freckles. Let your comfort level be your guide.

HAZARDS TO YOUR SKIN

First the good news: If we take real good care of ourselves, our skin—barring serious injury or a specific disease—will by and large take care of itself. Luckily for us, it's designed to do just that, and wonderfully so. Now the bad news: Many of us don't take real good care of ourselves! Junk food, smoking, alcohol, too much sun, too little sleep, exposure to pollution, and a host of other avoidable and unavoidable factors can compromise the health and looks of your skin.

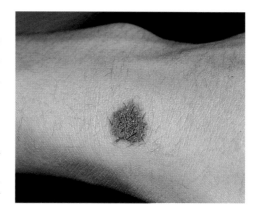

Above:
If you are concerned about an obvious birthmark or unsightly mole, consult a dermatologist.

The skin, you see, stands as not only the largest organ in the body but in many respects the ***most vulnerable*** as well. To give just one example: We all worry about the health problems that can be caused by air pollution once it reaches our lungs, but where do those pollutants land first? Our skin, of course! In fact, no other vital organ endures such constant exposure to the elements. No other organ is so directly subjected to traumatic injuries such as cuts, bumps, and scrapes, nor to the legions of viral, bacterial, and fungal nasties that would scare you half to

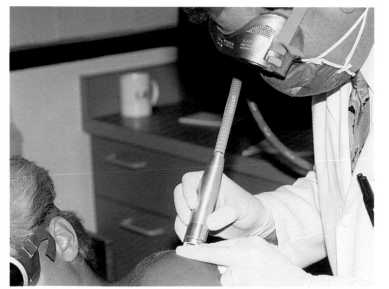

Left:
A dermatologist can remove a mole or birthmark with a laser.

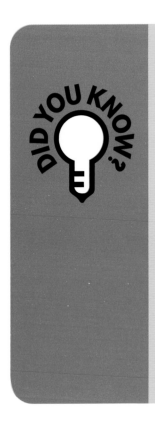

For ease of reference, most people refer to the skin as an organ, but it's really more accurate to identify it as an organ system that includes not just the flesh on our face and body, but also...

- Fingernails
- Toenails
- Hair
- Eyelids
- The thin, watery-looking mucous membrane covering the eyes
- The mucous membranes lining the inside of both the mouth and the nose

In subsequent parts of this book, you'll get some invaluable tips on manicures, pedicures, shampoos, conditioners, moisturizers, and more, because proper skin care doesn't begin and end with treatment of acne—it goes from head to toe. But don't you dare flip ahead; we have lots of important ground to cover first!

death if you saw them under a microscope the way a doctor or researcher does. And finally, no other organ must cope with the intensive use—and, worse, misuse—of the various cleansers, polishes, lotions, oils, and balms that have our medicine cabinets and cosmetics bags bulging to the breaking point. Our poor skin, in short, is *out there*, with nothing more to defend it than our own good sense and perhaps the ribbed cotton tank we picked up at the mall last week.

Just imagine: If we could mess with our liver and kidneys as easily and as often as we can our skin, how long do you think most of us would live? Our guess, we're sorry to report, is not very long at all, especially when you consider that some of us exercise sounder judgment in caring for a pair of expensive leather pumps than we do in caring for our skin. Would anyone in full possession of her faculties, for instance, take a perfectly good set of pumps to the beach for no other reason than to bake them in the August sun until they became dry, cracked, and discolored? Or smear them with dozens of different creams and powders in a misguided attempt to dress them up for a date? Of course not. Yet we routinely perform similar atrocities on our innocent, unprotected hides, without a second thought as to the long-term consequences. Go figure!

DON'T LET YOUR LOOKS GO UP IN SMOKE!

The general health risks associated with tobacco abuse—among which we may include chronic bronchitis, emphysema, heart disease, mouth cancer, throat cancer, lung cancer and problem pregnancies—are so well documented and so well publicized that we will not go into them here. Instead, we will touch briefly on how the smoking addiction harms your skin. To begin with, the nicotine in cigarettes causes your blood vessels to constrict, thereby reducing blood flow to your extremities, lowering the surface temperature of your skin, and dehydrating your epidermis. Since good blood flow is critical to both the color and texture of your skin, the lack of it results in a pasty, lifeless, grainy complexion, reflective of skin that has been starved of the nutrients, water, and oxygen a better blood supply would have provided. Smoking also exposes us to premature wrinkling by damaging the elastin fibers, which tend to become thicker and less resilient in people who smoke than in those who don't. Smokers, in fact, are many times more likely to suffer early or severe facial wrinkling than nonsmokers are. Finally, the very act of smoking itself does damage to the face and skin, even if we totally ignore the toxic effects of the poisons contained in the actual product. Every time you draw on a cigarette and exhale the smoke, you make a pronounced puckering motion with your lips and mouth. Smoke often enough and long enough, and this constantly repeated puckering will lead to the development of deep creases (called lipstick bleed lines) that fan out from the circumference of the mouth. Lines also typically radiate from the corners of the eyes in long-time smokers, possibly as a result of the continual irritation and facial tension caused by drifting fumes.

Smoker's face is a term used to describe the full, long-term impact of this incredibly nasty habit on the skin of your kisser—the pallid coloring, the rough texture, the creases, the wrinkles, the lines. If and when you are tempted to try a cigarette—or if you're already hooked, to light up your next one—we suggest you take a gander at the illustration on this page. Then ask yourself: Do I really want to look like this 15, 20, 25 years from now? We can assure you that many adult smokers now wish they had asked themselves that question, as well as several others, back when they first started.

THE LAST WORD

All of this brings us to one central point, and it's so important that we will set it off in capital letters and put a box around it so that you will hopefully never, ever forget it:

> NO ONE CAN DO AS MUCH TO PROTECT, BEAUTIFY, *OR DAMAGE* YOUR SKIN AS YOU CAN.
> TAKE CHARGE!

If you remember nothing else from this book, let it be the statement above. The bulk of our discussion from this point forward will be devoted to demonstrating how you can put that statement into everyday practice for a healthier, more beautiful you.

Right:
Take a look at your mom, grandmother, and aunts to get an idea of how you will age (but read on for tips on how to slow the aging process).

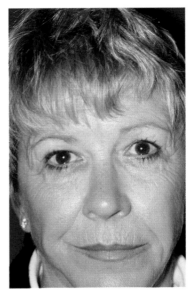
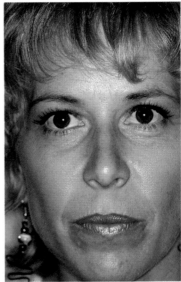

Derma...What?

You may have noticed that the words *dermis* and *dermatologist* sound a lot alike. Now, that's not too surprising since both derive from the same Greek root, *derma*, meaning skin.

A dermatologist, fittingly enough, is a medical professional who has successfully completed all the broad-based training in "conventional" medicine required to become a general practitioner (what you or I might call an *everyday physician* or *family doctor*), but with many additional years of specialized instruction exclusively in the skin. Odds are that most of us will need—if not now, then at some point in our lives—to visit a dermatologist's office, whether for care of problem acne, treatment of a troublesome cyst, removal of a birthmark, or cosmetic surgery of one sort or another.

Because far too many people still think of a dermatologist as someone who deals solely with acne and skin rashes, we've included a separate chapter (Chapter Ten) that provides detailed information on a pair of widely overlooked and generally misunderstood topics . . .

- The full variety of services offered by dermatologists today
- How to choose a qualified dermatologist who is *right for you*

Facts to Bore Your Friends With

The skin of an average human being covers an area of more than 20 square feet—about enough to make a good-sized tablecloth or a dozen small handbags!

Let's Take a Closer Look at Those Roots

We've already mentioned that the ancient Greek word for skin is *derma*. Its Latin equivalent is *cutis*. Many of the apparently difficult terms you'll encounter in biology class—and in this book—derive from one of these two root words. Here are just a few examples . . .

- **dermis**—the sensitive, vascular (or blood-supplying) middle layer of skin
- **epidermis**—the outer, nonvascular portion of the skin, which gets its name by combining the Greek *epi* (upon) with *dermis* (skin)

- **dermatologist**—someone who studies the skin and its diseases
- **dermatitis**—a general term that refers to inflammation of the skin
- **cuticle**—a word that, though actually synonymous with epidermis, is more often used to describe the thin, U-shaped sliver of dead skin at the base of the fingernails and toenails
- **subcutaneous**—the protective, insulating layer of fat beneath the dermis; also referred to as the *subcutis* layer in some sources

As for the word skin itself, that one derives from the Old Norse *skinn*, which sounds to us like it ought to be the name of an alternative band. Who knows? Could be it already is!

Quote Factory

If you wonder whether we're exaggerating about the effects of damage to the collagen and elastin fibers, just listen to how one of Shakespeare's characters describes it in *Henry IV*, Part 1:

My skin hangs about me like an old lady's loose gown.

Ouch! And the worst part is, that's precisely how it looks!

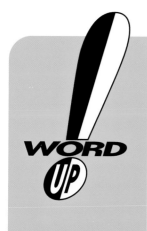

Just for fun, take a quick glance at the list of the scientific terms used in this chapter and see how many you can define now. If you can't remember one or two, simply thumb back through the text and look for the words we've italicized to refresh your memory.

- subcutaneous layer
- dermis
- collagen
- elastin
- epidermis
- keratinocytes
- melanocytes
- melanin
- dendrite
- dermatologist

END NOTE

1. For simplicity of presentation, we speak of the skin as having three layers, but to a biologist's or dermatologist's trained eye, there are many, many more than that. The epidermis alone, for example, displays three major strata, which can be further subdivided into some twenty remarkably thin (but still distinct) layers.

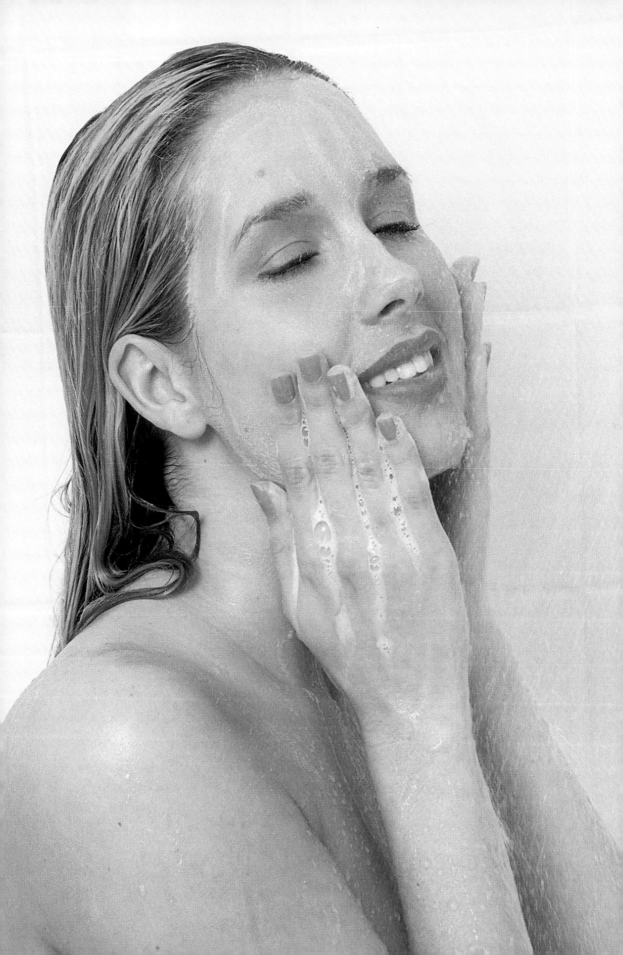

In Your Face!
Cleansers & Cleansing
for Best Results

We'd be the last people on the planet to suggest that cosmetics don't often work wonders to highlight your flattering features and help camouflage your flaws. However, there is one thing they simply cannot do: Give us the naturally clear, vibrant look that characterizes healthy, blemish-free skin at its best. Sure, we can salvage the appearance of dull, tired skin, to a point, with moisturizers and creams. And, yes, it's possible for us to conceal even the most persistent shine with just the right blend of blush, brush, and savoir faire. But, all else being equal, healthy skin translates to good-looking skin, and healthier skin to better-looking skin. Fortunately, we possess the power, by and large, to prevent or limit many of the factors that imperil skin health, and to promote many of those that sustain and enhance it, by doing nothing more than washing properly. Our thought for the day in this chapter, then, is *cleansing*.

IT ALL STARTS WITH CLEANSING

Proper skin maintenance begins and ends with that most basic of daily rituals—washing up, or cleansing, to use a term that more fully describes the complete process. Now, you may have thought that you had learned all you ever needed to know about this particular skill the day your mother first marched you to the sink and handed you a damp washcloth and a bar of soap. But in reality, cleansing the skin correctly isn't quite so simple as it initially appears, and just a few minutes of extra time and effort in the store, and at the bathroom sink each day, can pay surprisingly big dividends over time.

To wash more effectively, we need to learn exactly what happens when our skin gets dirty, and how to remove that dirt without irritating the skin or sapping it of necessary moisture. Though we will focus primarily on facial cleansing in this chapter, we will also touch briefly on body cleansing in places where that is relevant.

NOW GIVE US THE DIRT . . . *ALL OF IT*

In everyday usage, the word "dirt" conjures up mental images of the stuff we see in a flowerpot—chunks, clods, and granules, what a scientist or doctor would refer to as "particulate matter." The dirt found on our skin's surface, however, looks, feels and behaves quite differently from the garden variety dirt that feeds our mums and begonias.[1] It's more of a film or paste, a bit like the layer of oily scum you see on top of some roadside puddles, but thicker. This scuzzy coating occurs when the body's natural oils combine and chemically interact with impurities such as dust, grit, grime, bacteria, residual makeup, and our own dead skin cells. If the situation gets bad enough, a nasty compound of waste products builds up and coagulates, clogging our pores, inhibiting the operation of our oil and sweat glands, and interfering with the replacement cycle of live skin cells for dead ones. Once this happens, our body's natural oils deteriorate quickly and become contaminated, leaving us with a complexion that's dull, pasty, and lifeless if we have inherently dry skin, or greasy and slick-looking if we have oily skin. Nice, huh?

THE MARRIAGE OF SOAP & WATER

Since the dirt we've just described is *oil-based*, water alone can never be sufficient to cleanse it from the skin. Do you remember the last time you rinsed a frying pan that had a layer of cooking grease or vegetable oil on it? Unless you used some sort of soap or detergent, the water no doubt just beaded up and rolled off, leaving the grease right where it was before. Well, the same sort of thing takes place when we attempt to rinse oily dirt off our skin with mere water. Granted, rinsing *feels* delightfully refreshing and cleansing, especially on a hot day, but we shouldn't delude ourselves into viewing it as even a partial substitute for washing with both soap *and* water.

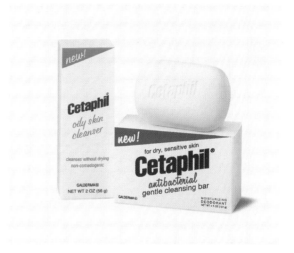

Soap and water form a magical combination because, in chemical terms, water requires an *emulsifier* to bind to dirt and actually remove it from the skin's surface. Though some other chemical compounds can also do the trick, soap remains the most effective, economical, and readily available emulsifier for the majority of skin types. When we apply soapy water to the skin, the soap attaches itself to the oily residue on the skin's surface and dissolves it to the point where a thorough rinsing can whisk away the accumulated crud.

Above:
Proper cleansing morning and night is essential for great-looking skin

If that were the full story, we'd stop right here and advise that you buy the strongest bar soap you could find. But there's a catch: Though stronger soaps attach themselves more securely to dirt, dissolve oil better, and therefore clean more thoroughly and efficiently than milder soaps, they are also apt to be more dehydrating and irritating to the skin. A very gentle soap, for its part, will generally leave your skin moister[2] and less irritated, but also less clean.

The Dope on Soaps

Thus far, we've been speaking as if there were but two families of soap in the world: the strong and the mild. But as those of

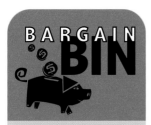

BARGAIN BIN

Some soaps melt very quickly once they become wet, while others are more durable. So if you're interested in saving some money, we recommend choosing a bar that stands up well to water. You'll find yourself buying new bars less often, and—as a bonus— wind up with less goopy residue in your soap dish.

us who have spent quality time in the health and beauty section know all too well, the actual number of choices is way big—and more than just a trifle confusing. What, for instance, makes traditional bar soaps different from detergent soaps? Medicated soaps from deodorant soaps? Or transparent soaps from liquid soaps? Is it necessary to use cleansing creams and astringents to get really clean? Or does simple soap and water suffice? Etc. Etc.

Now, on the one hand, the impressive variety of soaps, cleansers, and creams offered today is a real blessing in that we can fine tune our medicine chest to our skin type. But on the other, it creates the potential for *uninformed* consumers to commit serious skin care errors, usually without even realizing they're making poor decisions. To cut through the clutter and select the right products for us, we'll need to define a few broad categories of soap types and discuss the relative benefits and drawbacks of each.

Traditional Bar Soap

The first and most common type of soap we have already encountered briefly—traditional, opaque bar soap, also known as *milled* soap because it is physically pounded (or milled) into bars during production. Tallow and either animal salts or vegetable fats are the core ingredients in most opaque bar soaps, though some brands also add lathering agents and/or fragrances to make the final product more appealing to consumers. Soaps in this category are typically reasonably priced and do an excellent job of cleansing, but can be irritating to sensitive skin types or when we overuse them. People with oily, normal, or even moderately dry skin should be able to find a milled soap that not only suits their needs well but also saves them a sizeable chunk of change compared with more specialized products.

Superfatted Soaps

Superfatted soaps compose a second category. As the name suggests, these soaps contain additives such as lanolin and cocoa butter that give them a higher fat content than ordinary milled soaps—anywhere from three to eight times more fat, depending on the brand in question. Superfatted soaps were created to combat the oil-depleting effects of conventional bar soaps, which pull off not only dirt but also some of the natural oils that are meant to keep our skin nicely lubricated, supple, and smooth.

Do superfatted soaps achieve their goal? Well, yes and no. Yes to the extent that they tend to be gentler and less irritating to the skin; no to the extent that they generally cleanse less efficiently than old-fashioned bar soaps. In the end, it's a trade-off: If you have sensitive or relatively dry skin, a superfatted product may be just what you need. If, however, you have very oily skin and/or trouble with clogged pores, you'll probably want something that offers more robust cleaning action.

Transparent Soaps

Transparent soaps (you know, the ones that look so high-tech and, well, clean to begin with) form a third category, though they share a few similarities with the superfatted soaps we've just covered. Most brands in this category boast the high fat content of a superfatted soap, but also contain extra ingredients like glycerin, alcohol, or sugar, which makes them softer and more translucent (or see-through). Transparent soaps such as Neutrogena or Basis can be effective for those of us with oily, sensitive skin, since their higher fat content makes them gentler than toilet soaps, while their alcohol content allows them to strip off the excess grease that can clog the pores of our oil-rich skin. Conversely, these soaps are usually not a great choice for people with very dry complexions, because the alcohol in them can further dehydrate the skin, thus making a bad situation worse.

If you've ever used a bar of transparent soap, you may have been struck by the fact that it didn't produce a very generous lather. Most transparent soaps don't. Here it's worth noting that lather—or the lack of it—doesn't significantly affect a soap's performance as a cleanser one way or the other; it's there for aesthetic appeal only. For whatever reason, most of us seem to prefer a lot of lather, perhaps because it provides such a strong visual and tactile sense of cleanliness (My, just look at all those suds working away!).

Detergent Soaps

Detergent soaps—sometimes referred to as *synthetic* soaps or *soapless* soaps—are made from a mixture of petroleum products, fatty acids, and other chemical compounds. While the word "detergent" may lead you to believe that these soaps are somehow harsh or abrasive, most brands in this category are actually designed to be less irritating, less alkaline (that is, closer to the body's natural pH), and more richly lathering than regular bar soaps. The better detergent soaps, in fact, strike a nice balance between cleansing power and mildness, and thus often work well for normal, dry, and sensitive skin types. Finally, if you live in a hard-water[3] area, you will discover that detergent soaps offer an advantage over other bar soaps: Because they are oil-based, they rinse off cleanly and don't leave a soapy residue on your skin. Dove and Oil of Olay are examples of well-known detergent soaps.

Below:
Be sure to select the right cleansers for your skin type— many are available in both bar and liquid varieties.

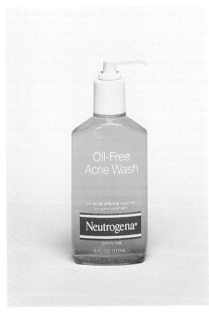

Liquid Soaps

Liquid soaps, which are becoming more popular by the day due to the convenience of the pump dispenser, do not form as distinct a category as, say, superfatted or detergent soaps. The majority of them, when all is said and done, differ little in terms of effectiveness from comparable bar soaps, despite the fact that they cost more than their messier rivals. The active ingredients in most liquid soaps are glycerin and detergent cleansers. As such, their suitability for various skin types is similar to that of the detergent soaps discussed above.

Medicated Soaps

Medicated soaps contain either prescribed or, as is more often the case, over-the-counter drugs to help treat specific skin problems like acne, eczema, and certain types of bacterial and fungal infections. Frankly, you should probably avoid such soaps unless one has been specially prescribed or recommended to you by your dermatologist. The reason behind this is that the medicine in medicated soaps

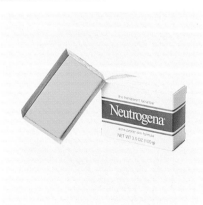

is almost always a *topical* agent, meaning that it needs to stay in contact with the skin for an extended period of time to work effectively. Unfortunately, the first thing we commonly do after applying soap to our skin is to rinse it off—*along with any medication it may have had in it*. If you saw someone put Clearasil on a pimple or Bactene on a cut (both topical medicines), then promptly wash it away, you'd no doubt think they were wasting both the product and their money. And you'd be right! So why do the same with your soap?

Soaps With Organic Ingredients

The manufacturers and marketers of soaps are smart people: They've learned over the years that today's health and beauty consumer has a positively insatiable appetite for novelty. Not surprisingly, they've acted on that knowledge by cooking up complete lines of product to feed our collective craving for the new and the exotic. The aggressive development and marketing of organic soaps, which feature "natural" ingredients like fruit juices, plant extracts, herbs, vitamins, and minerals, is a prime example of this trend.

While such soaps may strike us, at first glance, as somehow more wholesome or healthful than other kinds, the plain truth is that the organic ingredients in them are usually additives that have little or no therapeutic[4] value, nor any real bearing on the soap's cleansing capabilities. And even if these organic additives offered some benefit to the skin in their natural state—which, in many cases, is a doubtful proposition to begin with—their usefulness would be compromised almost entirely during the manufacturing process, in which soap ingredients are strained, mashed, sterilized, and blended beyond recognition. In this respect, most organic soaps are similar to most medicated soaps: They represent a premium-priced product that does no more for your skin than the modestly priced alternative that sits next to it on the drugstore shelf.

Deodorant Soaps

Deodorant soaps such as Lever 2000, Irish Spring, Dial,[5] and Safeguard seek to reduce or mask body odor. They accomplish this noble task by blending soap with antiseptics that control bacteria, perfumes that scent the skin lightly, or a combination of the two. As a rule, deodorant bars tend to be drying, and so serve better as body cleansers than as facial cleansers. In addition, the ingredients added to create the deodorizing effect can cause an allergic reaction in some people or act as an irritant to individuals with very sensitive skin. Despite these potential drawbacks, a deodorant soap can prove helpful if you experience problems with body odor. Just be sure to listen to your skin in the event you develop a mild rash or notice excessive dryness after bathing or showering.

Exfoliating Soaps

Exfoliating soaps are laced with very tiny flakes or grains of abrasive material that serve to chafe the skin lightly and thus scrape dead cells from the skin's surface. The most common exfoliate is pumice, or crushed volcanic rock, though it is not unusual to see ground walnuts, ground apricot seeds, cornmeal, and other substances (both natural and man-made) used as abrasive ingredients. The chief selling point of exfoliating soaps is that they are said to invigorate and renew the skin, rendering it clearer, smoother, and more vibrant than ordinary cleansers do. In theory, the process plays out like this: Once our dead, dried-up skin cells have been removed by the exfoliating soap, our dermis and epidermis are spurred into action and quickly increase the production rate of fresh, new skin cells. Because these cells are new, they are capable of holding and retaining more water than the dying and/or dead cells they replaced, which makes them plump up nicely to give us a firm, robust, glowing complexion.

While all of this is true to an extent, the argument for exfoliating soaps (and cleansers, which we will cover shortly) misses a couple of key points. First, the great majority of dead cells removed abrasively by exfoliating soap would have been shed naturally in a day or two anyhow, through the skin's own cellular replacement cycle. We simply don't gain that much in terms of time or cosmetic effect by hastening—and disrupting—the skin's own mechanisms for disposing of spent cells. And second, most abrasive soaps are just too rough and too drying to be used as everyday soaps. When overused, they can cause the skin to

become excessively dry, sometimes to the point of cracking and
peeling.

For these reasons, exfoliating
soaps—and abrasive cleansers in
general—are not recommended
for people with dry to normal
skin, sensitive skin, or anyone
with acne. Acne sufferers, in particular, can greatly aggravate the
seriousness of their condition
with facial exfoliates, and should
therefore avoid them entirely. If
you have an oily to very oily complexion, however, *occasional* use
of an exfoliating soap can make

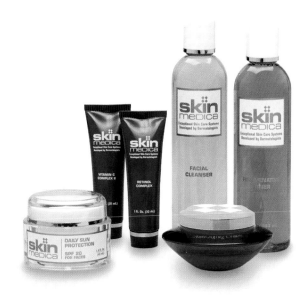

good sense because dead skin cells probably do tend to accumulate and close off your pores. But again, remember to exercise some restraint. The skin normally replaces cells over a 21-
to 28-day period. Give it time to do the work for you, and cut
back on your usage of exfoliating cleansers if your skin exhibits
a light rash, starts feeling itchy, or seems drier than usual.

Other Exfoliating Cleansers

Even if you don't wash with an exfoliating bar soap, you probably exfoliate your skin several times a day, often without realizing it. The use of a common washcloth, on a very basic level,
constitutes exfoliation of a gentle variety, and most washcloths
are textured for that very purpose. The loofah sponge we scrub
our back with also performs an exfoliating function, as does the
pumice stone that many of us use to grind dead skin from the
soles of our feet.

Nowadays, too, an increasingly broad selection of facial
cleansing products contain exfoliants as active ingredients. A
short list would include:

Scrubs

Scrubs are usually packaged and sold as creams, cleansers, or
lotions.[6] Like exfoliating bar soaps, scrubs rely on abrasive par-

ticles to remove dirt and excess oils, promote the sloughing off of dead cells, and prompt the production of new cells. But unlike most of the bars, these products typically contain emollients[7] and other ingredients[8] to make them milder and to help moisturize the skin. To get an idea as to whether a specific scrub will be compatible with your skin, you'll need to take a good look at the label. If the scrub is alcohol-based, you can be fairly certain that it will be somewhat drying, and for some skin types, irritating as well. If, on the other hand, the scrub is oil-based or water-based, it will most likely be milder but less efficient in cleaning your skin.

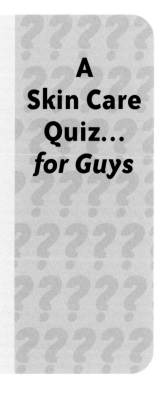

A Skin Care Quiz... for Guys

We gave you a quiz last chapter, so we figured it would be fun to have you give one to your favorite male friend(s) this time around. See how many of the following beauty terms he (or they, as the case may be) can define correctly, then grade according to the scale below.

- astringent
- T-Zone
- exfoliate
- pumice stone
- alpha-hydroxy acid
- loofah sponge
- aesthetician
- humectant

0 correct . . . Impressive, even for a male of the species
1 . . . Earth to [his name here], Earth to . . .
2 . . . Watches *way too much* ESPN
3 . . . Average, *real* average
4–5 . . . Slightly above average, but certainly nothing to be proud of
6 . . . A good showing; you could probably take him most anywhere
7 . . . Potential CEO of a major cosmetics firm
8 . . . He's been reading your magazines (again!)

Cleansers and moisturizers with alpha-hydroxy acid as an active ingredient

Alpha-hydroxy acid (often called AHA, for short) occurs naturally in everything from apples and oranges to cow's milk and wine. Over the past several years, AHA has been incorporated into a growing number of cleansers and moisturizers to serve as an exfoliant. Although they don't literally scrape off dead cells the way a sliver of pumice does, AHA achieves the same end by chemically irritating the skin, which speeds up the sloughing process and encourages the generation of new cells.

Facial masks

Often called cleansing or deep-cleaning masks, facial masks exfoliate the skin by pulling off dirt, oil, and dead cells after application and removal. There are essentially two types of masks: wash-offs and peel-offs. Wash-off masks are typically made from clay or clay-based ingredients, while peel-offs contain special chemicals that are designed to be applied as a cream, then dry to an ultrathin vinyl sheet that is later peeled away. In both cases, the principle at work is similar: We adhere the mask to the face for a half hour or so, during which time it dries, hardens, and contracts. This, in turn, creates a pulling effect that draws or lifts impurities and dead cells from the skin's surface.

As you can imagine, this drying process saps moisture not only from the mask, but from the face as well, which limits the usefulness of these products to oily skin types only. And even those of us with oily complexions need to be careful about *overusing* masks. If applied more than once a week, facial masks can stimulate the sebaceous glands to produce even more oil than usual.

Ultimately, though masks have a certain aura of pampered indulgence and idle luxury about them, they just don't do much by way of cleansing that other products can't do more cheaply and, in many cases, more effectively. So, unless you have an oily complexion and simply love the way your face feels after using a mask, you probably won't have to look too far to find a better and less expensive facial cleanser.

Astringents & Other Alcohol-Based Cleansers

Astringents are "soapless" cleansers that use either alcohol or, preferably, witch hazel to dissolve surface impurities from the skin. Unlike most other facial cleansers, astringents aren't designed to be rinsed off. Instead, the alcohol or witch hazel in them is meant to evaporate on the skin shortly after application, causing your face to feel temporarily cooler and tighter. This tightening or tingling sensation—which some manufacturers heighten with additives like boric acid, zinc, menthol, and eucalyptus—is a strictly aesthetic feature of the product, just as rich lathering is an aesthetic feature of some soaps. Your skin, then, will be no tighter or firmer after using an astringent than it was before, though it may be a good deal dryer if the brand you choose has a high alcohol content. Also, you'll want to be careful with astringents that contain the additives mentioned above: They serve no specific cleansing or restorative purpose, but can cause irritation or an allergic reaction in people with dry or sensitive skin.

Toners, bracers, skin fresheners, refiners,[9] and clarifiers are, with very few exceptions, alcohol-based cleansers whose ingredients and effects are so similar to those of astringents that it is difficult to make clear distinctions between them. The confusion created by this wealth of names is not only regrettable, but also sometimes misleading. Take toners, for example. Given the name, one would assume they firm up the skin the way exercise "tones" our muscles. But in reality, they do nothing of the sort. Like astringents, toners perform the less glamorous (but, in reality, no less useful) task of removing excess oil and residual soap from the skin, which is why so many women apply them after using an oil-rich cleansing cream or an especially "filmy" soap. The same holds true for bracers, fresheners, and clarifiers. These too, for all practical purposes, typically differ from astringents in name only.

One important exception: Some toners contain ingredients that can help prevent acne or combat the sun's harmful UV rays. Toners with AHA, like SkinMedica Acne Toner for instance, are designed to unclog the pores of acne-prone skin, while others with antioxidants are intended to fight premature aging and protect the skin from sun damage.

The best guidance we can give you if you wish to try an astringent—or an astringent-like cleanser—is to examine the list of ingredients carefully. Though most are alcohol-based, the amount of alcohol can vary widely from one brand or product to the next. In similar fashion, some astringents contain potentially irritating additives; others do not. Some attempt to counter the product's degreasing action with moisturizing ingredients; still others go the opposite direction by including exfoliating agents that strip even more oil from the skin. And if all of this sounds confusing, that's because it pretty much *is confusing*. As a general rule, though, look to see whether water or alcohol is the first ingredient listed. If water is first, the product is likely to be relatively mild and may be suitable for those with normal or combination skin. But if alcohol (or glycerin or acetone) is listed first, you're probably dealing with a strong, drying cleanser best used on oily skin only.

Cleansing Creams

Cleansing creams come in two basic styles: oil-based (or "tissue off") creams, and water-based (or "rinse off") creams.

Oil-based creams, like Pond's, are the older of the two kinds, and they rely on a mixture of oil, wax, and detergent to remove dirt, grease, and makeup from the face. Since these creams tend to be heavier and more oily than water-based varieties, the user must wipe them off with a tissue after application, then wash her face with a toner or astringent to clear away residual oils left behind by the product itself. Because a second step is required

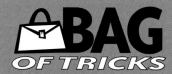

#!%*£§@# Mascara!

Nothing expands the vocabulary of even the most refined young lady quite so quickly as eye makeup that simply refuses to budge when we try to wash it off—a situation complicated by the fact that the eyelids and areas surrounding the eye are just as tender and touchy as they can be. For an answer that will help you come clean without extracting tears, we suggest you try one of the gentle eye makeup removers currently offered by most major cosmetics companies. Revlon and Clinique are two popular and widely available brands that we've used with good results, as are Cetaphil and Aquanil, both of which come highly recommended by most dermatologists. If even these gentle solvents irritate your eyelids or leave behind an oily film, you may have to switch mascaras. Look for a water-soluble—as opposed to waterproof—formulation that cleans off quickly and easily with a few swipes of a damp washcloth. Though you'll sacrifice some convenience (rain will be a pain, and you won't be able to wear it when you swim or play sports that make you perspire), at least you'll be able to get it off at the end of the day!

to clean the face thoroughly, oil-based creams are not a practical option as your primary cleanser. In practice, women use them almost exclusively as a means of gently removing makeup before the "real" cleansing begins.

Water-based creams, which are also sometimes referred to or packaged as washable creams, foams, gels, and gelees, behave more like soaps than like traditional, oil-based creams. Though all of them have the look and texture of a cream or lotion, their active ingredients are typically fats or detergents for cleansing, with oils added solely for softening. Even so, a conventional bar soap will generally outperform a water-based cream with similar active ingredients, in terms of sheer cleansing power. However, if you have very dry or sensitive skin, the mildness of a water-based cream can offer an attractive alternative to harsher or more drying cleansers.

As a final note on creams, bear in mind that even washable creams often contain a fair amount of oil.[10] That makes them an inferior choice for anyone with oily skin or acne, and a relatively better choice for dry and/or sensitive skin types. Just as dry skin normally reacts poorly to strong, moisture-draining products like exfoliating soaps and alcohol-based cleansers, oily skin ordinarily reacts poorly to mild, moisturizing products like superfatted soaps and cleansing creams. Ultimately, then, it pays to know your skin type, and to do your health and beauty shopping accordingly!

Choosing the Right Cleanser for You

By now, you realize that it is nearly impossible to make fair, even-handed comparisons between different brands or kinds of soaps and cleansers, inasmuch as the best item for you may be completely inappropriate for your neighbor across the street— or your classmate one row over.

So what's a young woman to do? That much, at least, is easy: Select the strongest soap or cleanser your skin type can handle, but don't get carried away. For those of us with extremely dry, sensitive skin, it could be that even the least offensive soap on the drugstore shelf is more than our skin can deal with. We may have to go the milder route of choosing a very gentle cleansing cream or lotion. For others, a stronger product will do. To figure out what's right for you, see your dermatologist, consult an aesthetician, or use old-fashioned trial and error by purchasing a variety of cleansers until you find one that cleans to your satisfaction but doesn't leave your skin feeling taut and dry. Since bar soaps are relatively economical and cleanse well, we suggest you start there, unless you know for a fact that your skin reacts badly to them.

One note of caution, however: Don't seek change solely for the sake of change or because you think another brand of soap may be sexier (or more feminine, or hipper) than one you've been using successfully for a number of years. If your current soap cleanses effectively, is affordably priced, and doesn't cause drying or inflammation, you're probably best served to stick with it rather than risk using an unproved product that may not agree as well with your skin. Save the experimentation and brand-switching for products that aren't performing as well as you'd like!

COMMON FACE-CLEANSING MISTAKES

You'd think it would be awfully difficult to mess up a task as basic as washing the face. After all, it's not as though we don't get plenty of practice! But scores of intelligent, well-intentioned people still manage to botch the affair—day after day, year after year. The four most common mistakes we've noticed are:

1. **Choosing the wrong cleanser.** Buy the wrong soap or cleanser and you're lost before you've even had a chance to start. It would be interesting to know just how many people with normal skin believe they have a dry complexion, when what they really have is a drying soap. Or how many women with only slightly oily skin are out there gleaming like Christmas trees because they wash with a thick, oil-based cream that's entirely incompatible with their skin. Probably more than we'd like to imagine. To keep this from happening to you, perform the skin test we've included in this chapter (pages 39-40), then pair your skin type with a complementary cleanser from one of the groups we've just discussed. If what you're using now seems a good match *and* works well for you, why then you're probably set. But if your current cleanser seems a bad match and your complexion is noticeably too oily or too dry, a change may well be called for.

2. Washing too roughly. For skin to stay soft, smooth, and supple, it must always be treated with tender loving care. That means: Don't yank it. Don't spank it. Don't push it around. Be nice. And above all, be gentle. Vigorous scrubbing and scouring may do great things to combat the built-up grease on a frying pan or the caked mud on your boyfriend's SUV, but then again, your face is not made of metal. Instead of slapping, scrubbing, and wiping, think in gentler terms like splashing, massaging (lightly, now!), and patting. Your skin is much less apt to become overly chafed and dry if you do. Skin that feels dry, tight, or rough after washing is a dead giveaway that you're working too hard, and perhaps damaging your skin in the process.

3. Washing too quickly. Washing your face shouldn't take more than 3 or 4 minutes, tops. Yet many of us are too impatient to devote even that miniscule amount of time to it! The argument against the "wham-bam" approach to washing is twofold: First, it doesn't afford our soap or cleanser enough time to bind to impurities and dissolve them; and second, we are likely, in our haste, to do a poor job of rinsing and may thus create a drying effect by failing to fully remove residual soap or cleanser from our face. It's likely, too, that rough washing often stems from hurried washing, which of course compounds both evils. So if you find yourself rushing along at the sink, just take a deep breath and remind yourself how much cleaner you'll be—and how much more refreshed you'll feel—for having washed your face gently and completely.

4. Washing too often. No doubt about it, we Americans are neat freaks through and through. And while our compulsion for cleanliness has its hygienic upside, it often causes us to wash (and bathe) more frequently than is altogether good for the skin. Two face washings a day ought to do the job for most young women: once in the morning on waking, and once at night before bed. If you play sports or work in an especially grimy environment like a fast-food restaurant, then a third washing before dinner or when your shift is over may be in order. But no more than that. Too much of the good thing called cleansing is a sure way to rob your skin of necessary moisture and leave your complexion dry, tight, and lifeless.

A SIMPLE, EFFECTIVE FACE-CLEANSING ROUTINE

This efficient, no-frills routine should not only clean your face thoroughly and gently, but also help to get you out the door on time.

- Moisten your full face from the hairline to the base of the neck by lightly splashing with lukewarm water or patting with a damp washcloth.
- Mix your soap or cleanser of choice with water until it lathers, then gently apply a nice, even coat to your face.
- Let the lather stay on your skin for 20 to 30 seconds to give it time to work. If, like us, you're the impatient sort, it wouldn't hurt to count out the seconds. Half a minute can seem an eternity when you're just standing there waiting!
- Rinse your face thoroughly by lightly splashing with warm (not hot) water.
- Pat (don't rub!) your skin dry with a fresh washcloth or towel.
- Repeat the entire process a second time, but with a cold-water splash when you rinse.

Those of us who use exfoliating bars, creams or lotions, by the way, need to be particularly gentle when applying the product to our face. The temptation, of course, is to actively "work" the cleanser into the skin with a forceful rubbing or massaging motion to help it get deep into the pores it's supposed to unclog. But as we've learned, this will only increase the abrasiveness and moisture-sapping effects of an already abrasive, drying cleanser. To be safe, use an extra light touch with exfoliating facial products, and be sure to keep them away from sensitive areas like around the eyes and just under the jawbone and chin. Here again, "elbow grease" is your enemy, not your friend.

MOISTURIZING—WITH & WITHOUT MOISTURIZERS

Throughout our review of cleansers and face cleansing, we've noted at several points that certain products can be drying to the skin. Indeed, the very act of washing the face is, to one degree or another, a drying process. What could be more logical, then, than to supplement our facial cleansing routine with a moisturizing cream or lotion? Shouldn't we do something to replace lost moisture and avoid the "dry, parched" skin the cosmetics ads warn us about? Surprisingly enough, the answer for most women 25 and younger is an emphatic "no!"

To understand why this is so, you need to realize that the skin derives its moisture from a mixture of water and *sebum*, the naturally produced oils of our sebaceous glands. Most younger women, as we've already observed, are fortunate enough to possess very productive sebaceous glands, which makes them less likely to suffer from the excessively dry skin that plagues so many of their elders. Consequently, it's rare for teenagers to have any practical grounds for using moisturizers of any sort, with the exception, perhaps, of those found as additives in sunblock or in very drying cleansers. Products whose primary purpose is to moisturize the skin, for the most part, belong almost exclusively in the cosmetics bags of women 30-plus.

Of course, it's true that a certain percentage of people are born with genetically dry skin and therefore may benefit from the use of moisturizers throughout their lives. But since this group forms a distinct minority, especially among teens, we've chosen to focus relatively less attention on cosmetic moisturizers, and comparatively more attention on ways our readers (of all skin types) can avoid losing surface moisture due to environmental factors and diet. Among these factors, we can include:

Air conditioning. Most of us switch on the AC in late spring and keep it humming all summer long without devoting a moment's consideration to how it works. As long as it's 72°F inside when it's 90°-plus outside, we are cool, content, and generally untroubled by the machine's internal workings. But you should be aware that *air conditioning constantly robs your skin of moisture*. Here's why: An air conditioning unit cools the environment around you—whether in the house, car, office, or classroom—by extracting warm, humid air from the immediate atmosphere and sending back dry, treated air in its place. When you work, study, watch TV, shop, or even just sit or sleep in an air-conditioned room, moisture is being pulled from the surface of your skin no less than it is from the air around you. (Most modern furnaces, too, pump out dry air unless they happen to be equipped with a humidifier.)

Now, it would be silly to suggest that you give up AC in the summer or the furnace in winter. We certainly wouldn't! But there are at least a couple of things you can do to prevent it from stealing more of your skin's moisture than is absolutely necessary. For one, take advantage of those cool, breezy days that occur every so often in summertime by shutting down the air conditioner and opening some windows. You—or your folks, if you live at home—will not only bring badly needed moisture into the house, but also save some money on the electric bill. A second trick is to keep a bowl of water near you whenever you're inside for an extended stretch. That way, the machine will drain more fluid from the bowl and less from your skin.

In the winter, humidify the air when the house is shut tight and the furnace is running full tilt. You can do this by either using your furnace's built-in humidifier, if it has one, or purchasing a free-standing, electric humidifier of the kind offered at most hardware or discount department stores, if not.

Exposure to the elements. Mother Nature, from everything we can tell, really has it in for the skin. The continual assaults of sun and wind in the summer, and cold, dry air in the winter, rob plentiful quantities of moisture from those of us who spend lots of time outdoors. In both cases, the culprit at work is evaporation, which dries out the topmost layer of the epidermis. This layer, known technically as the *stratum corneum*, is chiefly composed of dead cells that don't hold a great deal of moisture to begin with, but do provide a measure of protection for the plumper, moisture-rich cells below. When your face becomes chapped— whether from the effects of sun, wind, or cold—it's a sure sign that you should either be spending less time in the elements or covering your face more fully when you do. In situations where you cannot avoid being outdoors in extreme weather, we recommend a mild, moisturizing cream or lotion on

Below:
Whatever the weather, be sure to protect your skin from dehydration.

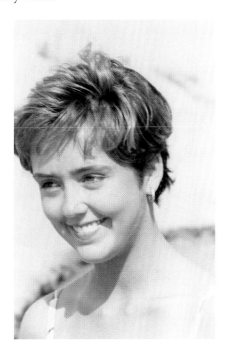

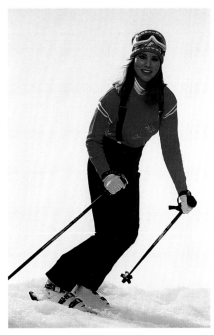

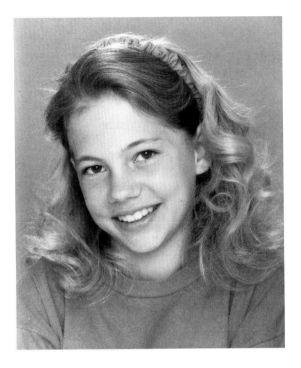

Above:
"Normal" skin like Shelley's is what we would all like to achieve.

the worst winter days, a sunblock with built-in moisturizers on nearly all summer days.

Not drinking enough water. Dietitians advise that we drink a minimum of eight 8-oz. glasses of water per day, and more if we're involved in physically intense activities that cause us to sweat a lot. But despite the clear guidelines, most folks don't come close to consuming as much water as their body requires for full hydration. This water shortage, of course, affects not only our internal organs but the skin as well. So lap up that H_2O! You'll get your eight glasses a day quite easily by having water with meals and using it—as often as possible—as a substitute for less healthy beverages such as coffee, soda, and caffeinated teas.

If you find that your skin is still bone dry—even after you've done everything within your power to preserve its natural moisture—we highly recommend two new moisturizers, both of which are dermatologist-tested and hypoallergenic: SkinMedica[13] Protective Day Wear Moisturizer for daily use, and Rejuvenative Moisturizer for overnight use. These are light, oil-free formulations that can help soften dry, chapped skin without leaving a thick, pore-clogging residue behind. The company has also come out with an excellent formula for those who suffer from eczema or rashes—SkinMedica Alpha-5 Cellular Repair Cream, which contains a blend of fatty acids, aloe vera, and vitamins to help treat and moisturize sensitive areas safely and effectively.

To apply any moisturizer, wash your face and hands first, but leave the face slightly damp. Then spread a thin, even coat over moist skin, using the product sparingly (too little is better than too much), with a gentle, wiping motion to achieve complete coverage. Don't cake the stuff on and—this is important—don't rub or massage it into the pores. Keep in mind that since you're counting on those pores to produce sebum, you can't afford to have them blocked up—even with moisturizer!

WE KNOW YOUR TYPE—OR DO WE?

Classifying skin by "type" is a very inexact science. Its terminology, though used freely and frequently by everyone from skin-care professionals to your Aunt Julie, is loosely defined and open to interpretation. Yet we need to classify, if for no other reason than to sort through the dizzying assortment of specially formulated cleansers, creams, and moisturizers the cosmetics industry has cooked up for different types of skin. The most common terms used to classify skin types are, of course, normal, oily, and dry.

Seems simple enough, at least on the surface. But it's wise to be careful before you accept the system whole and slot yourself into one category or another. So prior to launching into a description of the various skin types, let's first acknowledge a few weaknesses in the general way we talk about them:

1. **Your skin type is not etched in stone; it can change over time.** When hormones kick in during puberty, for instance, it's not at all uncommon for a child's dry to normal skin to become more oily due to increased activity in the sebaceous (or oil-producing) glands. That's why adolescents and teens suffer more from whiteheads, blackheads, and other forms of acne than the rest of the population. Conversely, most of us Mom and Pop types find that our complexions have gradually become drier as we've aged, necessitating changes in the way we wash and care for our skin. Your skin type can even change on a seasonal basis, especially if you live in an area that experiences dramatic swings in temperature and humidity from one season to the next. In the end, all of this should suggest that what works for you today may not be the answer ten years—or, for that matter, two months—from now. You need to be sensitive to that fact, and periodically check your skin for signs of change.

2. **Skin types within each category can vary widely.** Hey, if solving the riddle of skin care were as easy as identifying an individual's type and adjusting from there, everyone would glow, right? But the real world is much more complicated than the classification systems we try to impose on it. Consider, for

example, the hypothetical case of two cousins, each of whom possesses what could rightly be called "oily" skin. Couldn't we safely presume, seeing as how they both have oily skin, that the same soap or cleanser would work equally well for both? We could, perhaps, if they were identical twins; but otherwise, probably not. Let's say, again for the sake of illustration, that cousin A has moderately oily, nonsensitive skin, while cousin B's skin is extremely oily and sensitive. Those differences alone would force us to recommend a fairly strong bar soap for A that would likely prove too irritating for B's sensitive skin, even though her complexion is the more oily of the two. So while it's undeniably helpful to know your general skin type, realize that some products and practices that produce successful results for others in your group may not work as well for you.

3. Different areas of the skin can vary in type. If you read popular women's magazines or look closely at cosmetics ads, you've no doubt heard about the dreaded T-zone—a term used to describe the patch of skin that stretches horizontally across the forehead, and vertically from the bridge of the nose to the bottom of the chin. Since T-zone skin tends to be somewhat more oily than that of other areas of the face, a host of products and skin care regimens have been developed specifically for it. But despite all the attention focused on the T-zone, this same patchwork quality of alternately dry and oily spots can often be found in other regions of the face, and indeed across the length and breadth of the skin's surface. Truth be told, most of us possess **combination skin** to one degree or another, though we will reserve that term in our present discussion for people whose complexion displays *marked* differences outside the T-zone.

Below:
Poof! There you glow!
(Actually, looking this great
takes a little effort!)

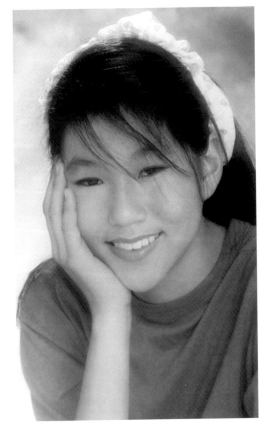

Testing for Skin Type

Despite these imperfections, classifying by skin type does allow us to deal with skin care issues intelligibly and to make suggestions that our readers can act on. For those suggestions to be useful, you'll need to first identify your skin type as precisely as you can. Let's run through each type and try to offer some pointers that should help you figure out where you fall in the dry to oily spectrum.

Step One: The Visual Inspection

The simplest and most obvious step in determining skin type is to (wonder of wonders!) look at the skin real close, using a magnifying mirror if necessary. But start first with an ordinary bathroom mirror. As you look at your face, check out your pores.

If you have **oily skin**, you'll observe large, open pores that are plainly visible to the unaided eye. Your skin, especially if you haven't washed in the past few hours, may even feel slightly oily to the touch. There is, of course, nothing wrong with being the proud owner of oily skin. It merely means that you, like many other women your age, are graced with active, hard-working sebaceous glands that will keep your skin supple and well lubricated, as long as you guard against oil buildup and subsequent blockage of the pores.

If you have **dry** skin, on the other hand, you will probably need to use a magnifying mirror to see your pores clearly. And because the pores of a dry-complected individual are so small and tightly bunched, that person's skin often gives the impression of being thinner, finer, and more translucent (or see-through) than oily or normal skin. Further, dry skin will almost always feel dry to the touch, even hours after washing.

Like oily skin, dry skin is neither a blessing nor a curse. If you have it, odds are you won't be plagued by an overly shiny T-zone, clogged pores, and certain forms of acne. However, you will want to take precautions against transepidermal water loss, which even in small doses can result in flaking, chapping, and irritation of your already dry skin. Some common causes of transepidermal water loss[11] are:

- use of an excessively strong and/or drying soap
- use of alcohol-based cleansers and cosmetics
- exposure to the elements
- exposure to air-conditioning (or forced-air heating)

Normal skin, since it stands between the relative extremes of oiliness and dryness, is perhaps the toughest skin type to define. To the naked eye, normal skin will appear moist and smooth, but not shiny or chapped, when viewed in the bathroom mirror. The pores, while visible without magnification, won't seem unduly large, nor will the texture of the skin strike you as particularly coarse or fine, as with other skin types. Normal skin looks—to be perfectly repetitive—normal, and so exhibits few or none of the more noticeable traits that help us distinguish very oily or dry complexions.

Step Two: The Paper Test

To confirm the outcome of your visual inspection, you should also try to gauge how oily or dry your skin is by testing it with facial tissue or lens-cleaning paper.[12] This test, too, is easy to conduct.

Begin by washing your face with a fairly neutral cleanser, that is, one that isn't exceptionally drying or loaded with moisturizers or added fats. A common bar soap or detergent soap should do just fine, as long as it's designed for general usage. Let your face recover from the washing for 3 to 4 hours, then cut your tissue or lens-cleaning paper into small squares. These will be used to test various areas of your face for oiliness.

The areas you should test include:

- forehead
- bridge of nose
- sides of nose
- cheeks
- chin

To test, hold a clean square of tissue or paper on each area for a count of ten. If your skin is naturally oily, nearly all of the squares will be oil-stained. If you have dry skin, all (or nearly all) of the squares will be unmarked. If you have normal skin, the squares applied to T-zone areas will show oil, while the others will be dry or show only the faintest trace of an oil mark. Combination skin, as might be expected, will render a mix of both oily and dry squares, particularly outside the T-zone.

BUYER BEWARE!

Most advertisers of health and beauty care items would like us to believe that the lustrous glow of the magazine covergirls is somehow locked within the featured product like a genie inside a lamp. Just take off the cap and . . . *poof*, there you glow! So, while there are literally thousands of fine, useful products on the market, it's smart to be skeptical when you read or hear ads about them. A soap or shampoo manufacturer, for example, may plug a new product as being "pH balanced," or claim that it "moisturizes while it cleans." What this usually means is that the product is nonalkaline and thus less prone to irritate your skin. So far, so good. But what the ad won't tell you is that the product's mildness has been attained at the expense of its cleansing power, which may or may not suffice to keep your skin as clean as you'd like it to be. Ditto for those soaps, usually targeted toward men, that make impressive statements about their cleansing properties but are silent on the subjects of moisture loss and possible irritation to the skin.

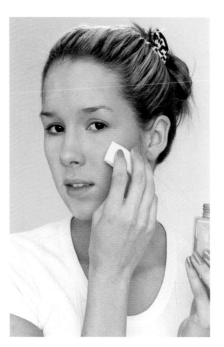

Below:
Choosing the right makeup formula for you skin type is just as important as choosing the right shade.

MATCHING YOUR MAKEUP TO YOUR SKIN TYPE

Nearly all of the principles that pertain to choosing the right cleanser for your skin type also apply to the sensible selection of makeup, despite the fact that the typical foundation or concealer contains literally hundreds of active ingredients, while the average bar of soap contains detergents and fragrances. To find cosmetics that will live compatibly with your skin on a daily basis, keep these general guidelines in mind when you shop:

- **Oil-based** formulations will coexist peaceably with dry skin most times, and with normal skin sometimes, but rarely, if ever, with oily or acne-prone skin.
- **Water-based** cosmetics (water appears first in the list of ingredients) are often good choices for people with dry to normal skin, since they can add a touch of lustre to an otherwise dull complexion.

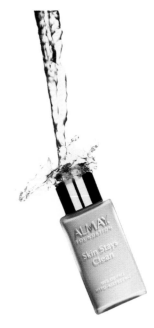

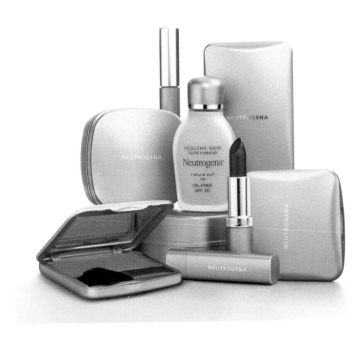

But if you have oily skin or trouble with acne, you need to know that these products aren't necessarily—or even usually—free of oil. Most often, they simply contain more water than oil, and thus may aggravate any existing problems you have with clogged pores.

- **Powder-based** formulations generally work well for those of us with normal to slightly oily complexions, as the powdery finish serves to tone down shine, especially in the T-zone. Conversely, they don't often make a good match for dry or chapped skin. Finally, powder-based makeup—like water-based makeup—may or may not contain oil, so you need to be sure of what you're buying if your skin is very oily or acne-prone.

- **Oil-free** makeup is best for oily or acne-prone complexions. Choose an alcohol-based or glycerin-based product if your skin responds well to astringent cleansers, a milder cream or lotion formulation if astringents tend to aggravate your acne or cause your skin to burn and redden on application.

END NOTES

1. You may argue that you've seen particulate matter covering your younger brother's skin after he's been to the park or played in a ballgame, but that is a separate issue altogether.

2. Don't be misled by soap ads stating that one brand or another will "replenish" or "restore" moisture to the skin. Any soap, no matter how gentle, actually *pulls* moisture (i.e., bodily oils) from the skin. As we've seen, it wouldn't work if it did anything else!

3. Water is said to be "hard" when it has a high mineral content. Though there is nothing essentially wrong or unsafe about hard water, it doesn't do a great job of fully dissolving soap film, which causes it to leave behind a soapy residue on the skin and in the sink after you've rinsed. You can solve the problem one of two ways: chemically soften or condition your tap water to reduce its mineral content, or use a detergent cleanser for washing. Either option should work just fine.

4. The word "therapeutic," when used by health and beauty care manufacturers, most often means "healing" or "restorative."

5. Hence the company's famous advertising slogan: "You use Dial. Don't you wish everybody did?"

6. A lotion, in most instances, is a watered-down version of a cream. The higher water content (and lower oil content) of a lotion will usually cause it to be less irritating and drying than a comparable cream, though it always pays to check labels to ensure that you're making a comparison between like products.

7. An emollient is an oil-based or fat-based ingredient that forms a barrier to seal in the skin's moisture. Some common emollients include petrolatum, lanolin, and mineral oil.

8. "Humectant" is another word you may come across when reading about moisturizing creams and cleansers. Humectants differ from emollients in that they draw moisture *to* the skin from the surrounding environment.

9. The group of astringent-like products sold as "refiners," "refining lotions," and "pore refiners" tend to contain more water than alcohol, and most often feature additives that may temporarily constrict the pores to make them appear smaller.

10. In fairness, we should mention that some *alcohol-free* gels currently on the market are suitable for nearly all skin types. However, you should look for one that contains a humectant (as opposed to an emollient) as the moisturizing agent if your skin is oily.

11. For more information on transepidermal water loss and how to prevent it, see pp. 34-35.

12. If you don't wear eyeglasses, lens-cleaning paper can be found in the eye care section of nearly any drugstore.

13. To order SkinMedica products, call 877-944-1412, or send email to info@skinmedica.com.

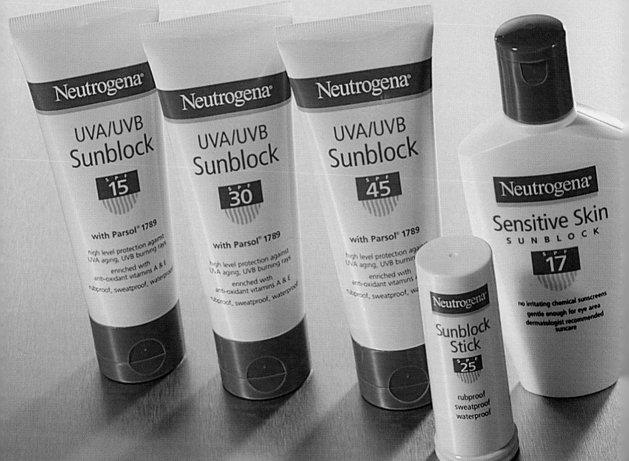

Sunsibilities:
Skin Protection Tips
& Sun Care Savvy

When you tan, you cook your skin. Simple as that. In fact, if it were up to us, we'd not only tell you that it's wisest to shun tanning under all circumstances, but also recommend that you keep your skin as completely covered as comfort allows on sunny summer days. But being realists, we know that the lure of the sun's warm rays and the promise of a hot, honey-brown complexion are sometimes too tempting to ignore, especially when swimsuit season rolls around and your legs are still as ghostly white as the snow that kept you indoors all winter. And then, too, so many of the activities that make free time worthwhile take place outdoors, so getting some amount of sun is almost inevitable. Tennis, softball, soccer, skiing, swimming, boating, picnics, and scores of other essentially healthy diversions are, we must admit, best enjoyed on bright, sunny days. So the question is: If we must expose ourselves to the sun, how can we do so in a manner that strikes a sensible balance between the lifestyle we want now and the problems we'd prefer to avoid down the road? To arrive at an answer, we need to start by analyzing the nature of sunlight, and how it alters and affects the skin.

SHEDDING LIGHT ON . . . UV RAYS

The sun emits a broad range—or spectrum—of light rays that vary in length and intensity. For our purposes here, the ones that matter most fall into the *ultraviolet* portion of the spectrum. These rays, usually called UV rays, are of intermediate (or medium) length, meaning that they occupy the segment of the spectrum between the longer rays that produce visible light and the shorter rays (known as X rays) that are not only invisible to the naked eye, but also extraordinarily powerful. Like X rays, some light rays in the UV spectrum are invisible and deceptively intense. When most of us hear the word "radiation," for example, we think of nuclear bombs and poisonous mushroom clouds. Yet we live with—and expose ourselves to—a steady stream of radiation every day in the form of sunlight.

UV light itself is broken down into three types by scientists who specialize in this sort of thing: UVA, UVB, and UVC. Thankfully, most UV rays, and all UVC rays, never reach the earth. The ozone layer of the atmosphere filters them out, thus saving our skins in the most literal sense of the phrase.[1] However, more than enough UVA and UVB rays sneak through the ozone to cause considerable damage to unprotected skin.

In the short term, this damage manifests itself as tanning or burning of the skin. UVA rays account for tanning, while UVB rays cause burning. Now, it would seem logical to conclude that UVA light is somehow less harmful than UVB, given that a sunburn creates so much immediate discomfort and produces such visibly dramatic evidence of injury. But as is so often the case in scientific matters, the apparently obvious, commonsense conclusion turns out to be . . . DEAD WRONG!

UVA & Tanning

Although UVA light doesn't burn the skin, it does penetrate more deeply than UVB light—straight down to the dermis, in fact. Its most immediate effect is to stimulate increased melanin production, resulting in the darkening or browning of the skin we refer to as "tanning." Just as a viral infection prompts the swift production of antibodies by your immune system so you don't catch a specific virus again, so too UVA radiation spurs the production of melanin by your melanocytes as a defense against additional UV exposure.[2] Far from being a sign of robust health or vitality, a really dark tan indicates that you've forced the skin to protect itself against an unwelcome invader with a heavy dose of pigmentation. At this point, some damage has almost surely been done, and your body is telling you in a very graphic way that it has had more sun than it can comfortably handle.

UVB & Sunburn

UVB rays, for their part, are less prevalent in sunlight than UVA, but possess some unique characteristics that make them even more dangerous to skin health. In contrast to UVA, UVB light does the majority of its dirty work on the epidermal (or outermost) layer of the skin, where it burns up keratinocytes (i.e., epidermal cells) and thus causes the familiar reddening and blistering we associate with sunburn. When you flake or peel after a long afternoon at the beach, then, your skin is simply sloughing off all the dead cells you've killed that day.

The burning process—and these are **real** burns, no less than if you had momentarily held a lit match to your face or scalded your back with boiling water—takes place in two distinct stages. The first stage, characterized by inflammation and a reddish cast to the skin, crops up just after exposure, then seemingly disappears after you've been inside for a while. This represents your body's initial attempt to combat the burn. But just when you think you might have escaped serious harm, the sunburn returns with a vengeance, usually 3 to 4 hours after exposure, then worsens over the next 24 hours. If you've experienced a relatively minor burn, the burned areas become pink and tender. However, if you've burned yourself badly, the injured regions turn deep red, blister, and flat out hurt. In extreme cases, the burned skin may literally feel hot to the touch even hours later.

Taking the Sting Out of Sunburn

Of course, the ideal remedy for a sunburn is NOT TO GET ONE IN THE FIRST PLACE. But in the real world, sometimes even the most conscientious of us manage to get burned. When that happens, your most immediate goals are to *reduce inflammation*, *restore moisture*, and *soothe the skin*. To do so, you should . . .

- **Get (and stay) out of the sun.** Sure, we could explain, but . . . *Duh!*
- **Apply a cold compress to the burn.** Whether you use the old-fashioned approach of wrapping ice in a washcloth or towel, or use one of the newfangled chemical compresses or ice gels, the idea here is to minimize swelling and provide some relief to the scorched area. But no matter how you go about it, be absolutely sure that your compress is as clean and sterile as you can make it, because burns (of any variety) are extremely susceptible to infection. Apply the compress as soon as possible after you first notice the burn, and keep it on the affected area for a solid 15 minutes. Repeat this process at least three times a day until the burn is no longer sensitive to the touch.
- **Apply a moisturizing cream or lotion** to the affected area after each cold compress, to relieve dryness and keep the wound lubricated.
- **Shower in cool water** until the burn heals. If you usually prefer to bathe, we recommend that you temporarily switch to showers until your skin has healed, to reduce the risk of infection.
- **Take aspirin** (or a nonaspirin, over-the-counter pain reliever like Ibuprofen) in recommended doses for short-term relief from discomfort.
- **See your doctor or dermatologist immediately** if the burn persists longer than a week, blisters badly, or becomes infected at any time.

The Long-Term Forecast

The short-term effects of overexposure to the sun, painful and unattractive as they may be, pale in comparison with the long-

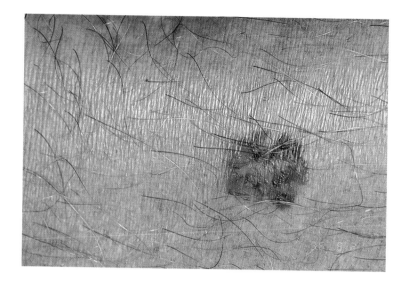

Left:
This seemingly innocent little spot is a melanoma—a skin cancer that can be deadly.

term effects. That's because **sun damage is cumulative and, what's worse, largely irreversible**. Damage builds up slowly over time, and since most of it occurs below the surface, doesn't become noticeable until a crisis point has been reached or surpassed. In this respect, people who habitually take too much sun are a lot like smokers: They may be perfectly well aware of the dangers of their behavior, but the lack of any immediate sign of trouble lulls them into a false—and all too often life-threatening—sense of security. This illusion, as you can imagine, is typically shattered the day they walk into a doctor's office and learn they have a deadly form of skin cancer.

So what are these effects that mount and compound through the years? Let's begin in the dermis. Here, prolonged and repeated exposure to the sun affects several key structures. We've already noted in Chapter One that too much sun—specifically, UVA rays—results in crippling of the collagen and elastin fibers that keep the skin tight, resilient, and free of wrinkles. Once these are shot, you're facing a lifetime of loose, puckered, wrinkled skin that only very extensive cosmetic surgery can even partially repair. Damage to the melanocytes also frequently occurs, and ultimately finds expression in blotchy pigmentation, the formation of moles, and the development of age spots (patches of permanently pigmented skin), all of which are red flags that you need to (a) start staying clear of sunlight *now*, and (b) see your dermatologist *immediately*. In the epidermis, UV light exposure stretches and dilates the tiny capillaries that carry vital nutrients and oxygen throughout the surface layer of the skin. In time, a weblike pattern of broken blood vessels forms just beneath the skin's surface, causing a condition commonly known as *spider veins*.

SKIN CANCER: BY THE NUMBERS

The worst possible outcome of long-term overexposure to the sun is, of course, skin cancer. We know of three types directly linked to sun damage (these types of skin cancer may occur on any part of the skin):

- basal cell carcinoma, which chiefly affects facial skin
- squamous cell carcinoma, which primarily attacks the head, neck, hands, and legs
- melanoma, which can establish itself anywhere on the body, but is most often found on the back or on the back of the legs

Basal cell carcinoma ranks as the most common form of skin cancer, accounting for some 80% of new cases. But of the three types, malignant melanoma stands as the most deadly variety by far. If not treated early on, it kills more than half the people who develop it within 3 to 5 years. And, though melanoma accounts for just 4% of new skin cancer cases, **it is now discovered more frequently in women aged 20 to 30 than any other form of cancer—skin or otherwise**.

In America alone, one million new skin cancer

Below:
Potentially dangerous moles should be removed by a physician and sent to a pathologist for evaluation.

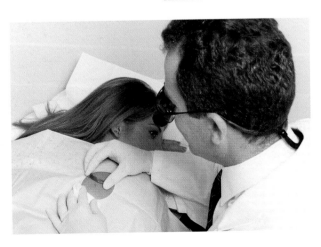

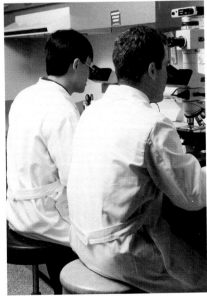

cases will be reported this year, many involving people who would have otherwise enjoyed a fairly clean bill of health. Consider, too, that recent statistics tell us that one in every five U.S. citizens will contract some form of skin cancer during their lifetime, and that one in eighty-four will develop melanoma.

Despite these sobering numbers, there is at least a little good news to share. For one, public awareness of the dangers posed by skin cancer is at an all-time high, and is steadily becoming more widespread. Second, most skin cancers can be treated successfully if they are detected in their earliest stages. And last, proper use of modern sun protection products, combined with sound judgment, should allow the vast majority of us to enjoy the outdoors fully *and* safely on all but the most blazing days.

A CLOSE LOOK AT SUN-DAMAGED SKIN

For some of us, the desire to tan can overcome even our worst fears about the physical damage caused by UV exposure. We reassure ourselves with thoughts like, "Heck, a half hour won't kill me." Or, "I never peel, and my Mom's skin looks great, so I must have good genes." Or, "I'll get my base first, then start using sunscreen." But sooner or later, continual UV exposure leads to permanent sun damage, and permanent sun damage

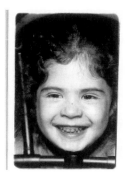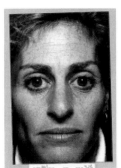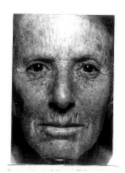
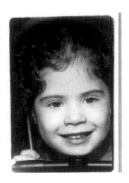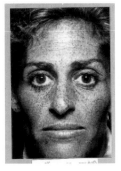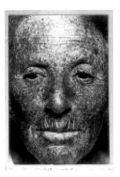

Left:
Examples of Sun-Damaged Skin.

Skin damage from exposure to the sun can be shown using an ultraviolet camera. The top three images were produced with a regular camera, and the bottom three were produced with an ultraviolet camera. The left two images show minimal sun damage, the middle two show moderate sun damage, and the right two are examples of severe sun damage.

Right:

This photo shows the skin on the face and the underside of the arm of the same woman; notice the sun damage on the face.

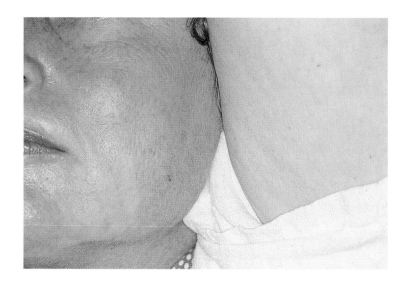

leads to skin so vile an alligator wouldn't be caught dead in it. We joke to keep things light, but it truly is heartbreaking to see what can eventually happen to the appearance of a woman whose skin has been ravaged by the effects of *photo-aging*, the term used by dermatologists to describe the effects of serious, long-term sun damage.

Photo-Aged vs. Healthy Skin

In healthy skin, the cells fit together in a nice, tight, interlocking pattern, much as the pieces in a new jigsaw puzzle snap together firmly when you first take them out of the box. Such cells—again, like new puzzle pieces—are flat and smooth, with crisp, clean, unfrayed edges. Sun-damaged (or photo-aged) skin, by contrast, resembles one of those puzzles you've taken apart and put together a zillion times. Though the pieces, as a whole, still form a larger picture, each one is now thick and rough-edged from years of hard use, resulting in a loose, mushy fit. Skin damaged in this manner has a granular, leatherlike texture that is visibly coarser than the smooth, almost seamless surface presented by undamaged skin. To gain a sense of the difference in texture and appearance, take a gander at the photo on this page, which shows moderately sun-damaged skin from a 40-year-old woman's face. Can you imagine how much younger this woman would look today if she had protected her face as thoroughly as her underarm over the years?

And this lady's skin isn't in exceptionally bad condition for her age! Severely photo-aged skin is, to put it bluntly, an ugly sight to behold: Beyond the rough, pebbly texture we've just described, it typically exhibits:

- a dull, lifeless complexion—in light skinned people, you'd probably say the look was pasty or sallow; in darker skinned whites and in blacks, ashy or muddy
- blotchy coloring, age spots, moles, and yellow, pimple-like eruptions, all of which signify irreversible damage to the skin's pigment-producing cells, and in many instances the presence of skin cancer
- a loose, wrinkled and often puckered appearance, stemming from worn out collagen and elastin fibers

The Critical Years: Age 20 and Under

Right now, dear reader, you are making critical decisions that will not only significantly raise or lower your risk of developing skin cancer, but also shape your looks for the rest of your life. Every piece of current medical research suggests that our first twenty years pretty much dictate what will eventually happen to our skin as we age. Now, this fact counts as neither good news nor bad news, in and of itself. It all depends on YOU. Regular use of sunblock before age 18, for example, can slash your skin cancer risk by as much as 50%, plus help your skin stay supple and smooth. Start even earlier, in childhood, and the risk reduction factor plummets to nearly 80%. But, on the other hand, research

Left and below:
The regular use of sunscreen early in your life is critical if you want to have beautiful skin throughout your life.

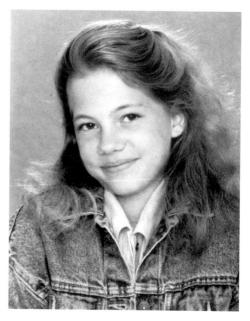

also indicates that early overexposure to the sun compromises skin health and raises your cancer risk to a far greater degree than overexposure later in life. So the choice is yours: You can set yourself up to be a haggard-looking and potentially cancer-ridden adult. Or you can do a few simple things correctly now—and probably wind up looking younger than your classmates and friends for years to come.

The right choice seems obvious to us, and we're sure it does to you, too. Fortunately, turning that choice into reality requires nothing more than acquiring the knowledge necessary to protect yourself from the sun, then cultivating a few good habits based on that knowledge. We call the whole package *"sunsible living,"* and it begins with understanding your own susceptibility to sun damage.

HOW *SUNSITIVE* ARE YOU?

Though everyone needs to protect themselves against UV radiation, there's no getting around the fact that some people tolerate the sun better than others. Blacks and dark-skinned whites, as you might have guessed, are significantly less prone to sunburn than their light-skinned neighbors. Likewise, people with naturally dark hair and dark eyes tend, on the whole, to weather the sun better than those of us with lighter features. To help you determine if you fall into an especially high-risk category, we've listed below several of the factors and physical traits that have shown a high correlation to the incidence of skin cancer.

Below:
How "sunsitive" are you? Fair-skinned types are more sensitive to the sun, but we all need protection.

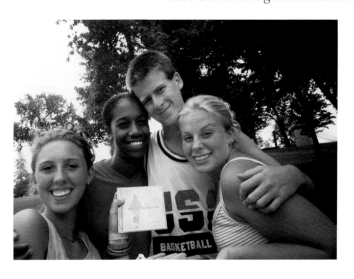

This doesn't mean that if many (or even all) of them apply to you that you will someday inevitably suffer from skin cancer. Nor does it mean that you are under no risk whatsoever if none apply. The list should, however, give you a sense of your relative capacity to take sun, and alert you to some of the more dangerous warning signs of sun damage. That much said, the likelihood that you will suffer from skin cancer is higher if you have:

- fair skin
- freckles
- a large number of birth moles
- several particularly large moles
- moles that are growing, changing shape, crusting, or bleeding
- light-colored eyes, such as blue, green, gray, or hazel
- light-colored hair—blondes and redheads, by the way, are 2 to 4 times more prone to skin cancer than the general population
- a tendency to burn rather than tan
- a tendency to peel and/or blister when you burn
- a tendency to freckle when exposed to sunlight
- a family history of skin cancer
- a job or lifestyle that often exposes you to excessive UV radiation

Below:
This abnormal mole (A) resulted from hours in a tanning salon. The skin is shown immediately following removal by a dermatologist (B), and 1 year later (C); the mole is gone and only the barest trace of a scar remains (the square patch next to the mole is where a tattoo was removed by a laser).

KNOW YOUR MOLES!
Part 1: Mole Tracking

As you can tell from the list above, moles often indicate that sun damage has occurred. Now, the presence of a few birth moles is no big deal: If you have fewer than five or six, and they are small and symmetrically shaped, you probably have little reason to worry. If, however, you start noticing new moles or begin to see changes in the ones you've had from birth, it could be an early warning sign of skin cancer or a related skin disease. So it pays to know your moles. Unfortunately, moles in inaccessible places like your back, buttocks, and hamstrings can easily go unnoticed, as can seemingly minor changes in the moles you already know about.

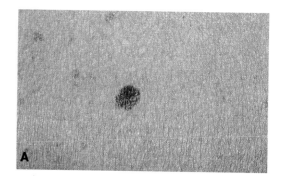

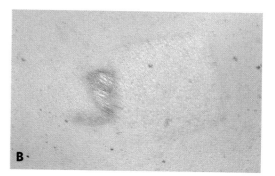

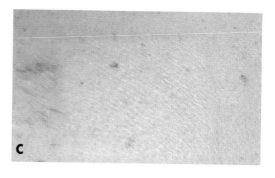

Dermatologists nowadays address this problem through a wonderfully simple and effective process called *mole tracking*, which involves taking photos of the moles you currently have, then noting their size and shape at the time of your visit. On subsequent visits, your doctor (or one of the nurses) does a thorough inspection of your full body to spot new moles, and also carefully re-measures your existing moles to make sure that none have grown or changed since the last mole tracking was done. If changes have taken place, new photos are taken and your file is updated with the new information. It's a quick, painless way to monitor skin health—and one that could help save your life should you ever begin to develop skin cancer. Needless to say, we recommend it highly.

Part 2: Self-Examination

Between doctor's visits, you should keep tabs on your moles and monitor your overall skin health through self-examination. Medical experts, in fact, now advise that we self-examine our skin on a monthly basis. Fortunately, this self-exam is easy to conduct and can be performed in the comfort and privacy of your own home. To perform one on yourself, use a full-length door mirror to inspect the front of your body, and a small, hand-held mirror to check tight spaces or hard-to-see areas like the back of the neck, the shoulders, armpits, back, and buttocks. You'll want to adopt a routine that ensures inspection of your entire body. So take a logical starting point, such as the soles of your feet or the top of your head, then methodically work your way up or down, as the case may be. Be sure to observe all skin surfaces on both the front and back of your body, including the scalp, the spaces between your toes, the skin behind your ears, and other regions where the light of day does not ordinarily shine. A thorough exam can be completed in just 5 to 10 minutes, and since any changes you observe

Below:
Self-examination for moles doesn't end with visible skin. remember to check your hairline and other hidden areas.

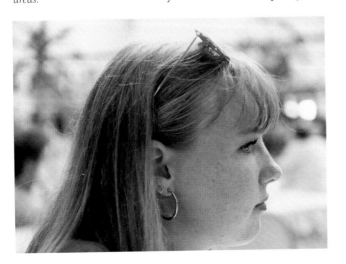

are likely to be subtle, this is the type of task that's best done slowly and carefully. As the saying goes, "work as if you were being paid by the hour."

A, B, C, D Warning Signs

We've already talked quite a bit about what ought (and ought not) to concern you in terms of the outward appearance of moles specifically, and of your skin in general. To keep the most significant warning signs clear in your mind, just think of the letters A through D as an acronym for:

asymmetrical moles . . . that is, moles that are unevenly shaped

border irregularity . . . or moles with notched, fuzzy-looking, or ragged edges

color . . . as you'll recall, uneven or blotchy color is worrisome, because it indicates that melanin is not being distributed as uniformly and consistently as it should be

diameter . . . a mole with a diameter that exceeds 5 millimeters needs to be checked, as does a mole that is changing in any way

TANNING: THEN & NOW

Historically speaking, our love affair with tanned skin is a fairly recent development. As a matter of fact, it wasn't until the early part of the 20th century that a tan was considered at all desirable. Prior to, say, 1920, tanned skin meant that you worked in the fields and occupied a relatively low rung on the social ladder. The land-owning rich, even if they happened to be sportsmen or nature lovers, viewed pale skin as a mark of wealth and distinction, and so took great pains to protect themselves from the blistering effects of the sun. When a well-to-do woman of the late 1800s went on a picnic, for example, she typically donned a full-length dress, buttoned it all the way up to the neck, then topped off the look with a broad-brimmed hat and parasol for added protection.[3]

Attitudes—and consequently fashions—began to change rapidly after the First World War. By that time, the Industrial Revolution had moved millions of manual laborers from sun-drenched fields to dark factories. The rich, along with the growing middle class, flocked to the outdoors in greater numbers than ever, and wore skimpier clothes[4] when they did. Tanned skin, once the tell-tale sign of rural poverty, had almost magically become symbolic of affluence and leisure. These perceptions continued and flourished in the decades that followed,[5] and it has only been in the past ten years or so that tanning has begun to lose some of its undeserved lustre. Nowadays, at least, public awareness of the threat posed by skin cancer has widened by leaps and bounds, and trendsetters (including top fashion models like Kate Moss and celebrity entertainers like Madonna) have been steering society away from the notion that tanned skin is somehow more appealing or sexier than a paler look. If nothing else, the fact that people now go to the drugstore to purchase sunscreen and sunblock, as opposed to the tanning oils they bought not so very long ago, illustrates that constructive changes in attitude and behavior are taking place, perhaps faster than we realize. Who knows? We may well go down in history as the last generation to find tanned skin attractive. Now *that* would be progress!

"Model" Behavior

The ideal role models for sun-smart skin care are probably waltzing down a runway somewhere in Paris or Milan as you read this book. Surprised? Well, you shouldn't be. Women whose livelihood depends on beautiful skin understand better than the rest of us that too much sun is the fastest route to prematurely aged skin, and for them at least, to the unemployment line. As a result, you won't find many successful models on the beach—even for a photo shoot—without sunblock, UV-filtering sunglasses, and a cover-up to throw over their swimsuit during the hours of the sun's peak intensity. The cast of the popular TV show, *Baywatch*, for example, uses gallons of sunscreen every week.

Truth be told, most models these days actually prefer an artificial, cosmetic tan to the real thing. The latest self-tanning lotions, which are vastly superior to what was being offered even just a few years ago, allow them to achieve a tanned look without risking the unavoidable skin damage and potential burning and peeling that make old-fashioned sunbathing such an iffy and dangerous proposition.

Peak UV Intensity: How It Works, What It Means to You

The intensity of the UV radiation you're exposed to at any given time and place depends on (1) the distance between you and the sun, and (2) the angle at which the sun's rays must travel to reach you. In basic terms, the shorter and more direct the hit, the greater the UV exposure. Even slight differences in distance and angle can produce drastically different results. Have you ever noticed, for example, how

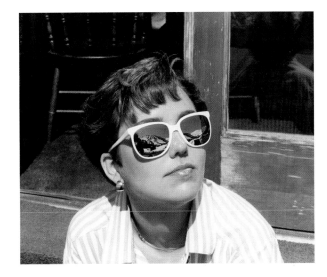

Above:
Sunscreen and sunglasses are essential at high altitudes.

much more quickly and severely you burn on your nose and forehead than on your legs? On your shoulder blades, as opposed to the small of your back? Skin sensitivity, of course, accounts for some of these discrepancies, but much of the reason your head, neck, and shoulders are so vulnerable to burning is that they usually receive the full force of the sun's radiation sooner and more directly than the rest of your body.

Since distance and angle combine to determine the relative intensity of sunlight, it's helpful to understand the factors that influence both. There are several, among which we can include:

- **Proximity (or nearness) to the equator:** UV intensity, obviously, is greatest at Equatorial latitudes, and gradually diminishes as you approach the North or South Pole.
- **Altitude above sea level:** The higher you climb, the more intense the sun's rays are, at a rate of about 4% more exposure for every additional 1,000 feet of altitude. This is an important nugget of information that some snow skiers and snow boarders fail to consider when they take to the slopes without sunblock on bright winter days. Backpackers and mountain climbers also need to make added sun protection part of their planning for every ascent—even if the elevation involved isn't that high. You don't have to scale Mount Everest or hike the trails to the top of Pikes Peak to burn badly at high altitudes.

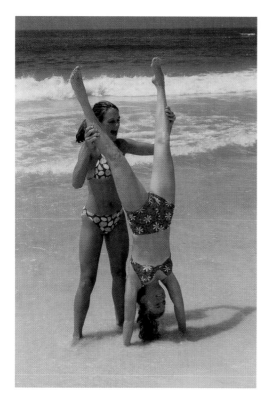

Above:
The beach is fun, but best enjoyed during "off-peak" hours.

• **Season of the year:** Summertime (surprise! surprise!) means more direct exposure, no matter where you live. And though common sense dictates that you take *extra* precautions during the warmest months of the year, don't assume that you can disregard UV protection throughout the fall and winter. Cool temperatures can mask the sun's true intensity, and snow-covered ground often acts as a reflector to give you a double dose of UV exposure. (Concrete and sand, by the way, also reflect UV light, and can leave you scorched in the strangest places if you're not careful. Burns under the armpits, along the calves, and at the back of the knee are not unheard of for this very reason. Ouch!)

• **The time of day:** The sun gives us its strongest blast of radiation at 12 noon, but anytime between the hours of 10 AM and 3 PM qualifies as a peak intensity period, by our reckoning. These hours are best spent indoors if at all possible, which isn't nearly so difficult or annoying as you might initially think. There's no need to, say, skip your daily run; just reschedule it for early morning or late afternoon, or find an indoor track if changing the time is an issue. You'll not only dodge the kind of intense UV exposure that can take years off your skin's life, but also get a better, more comfortable workout for having avoided the worst of the midday heat.

Ozone Alert!

Many local weatherpersons now issue "ozone alerts" on the evening news. Alerts are typically issued for summer days when high heat, high humidity, and excessive pollution combine to make the air difficult to breathe for those with heart or respiratory problems. And guess what? Those same atmospheric conditions also magnify the harmful effects of UV exposure. So if you hear an ozone warning during the weather forecast, don't think it's just for people with pacemakers and asthma inhalers. Take the meteorologist's advice, and stay inside until the air clears.

Don't Expect Protection From . . .

- **Cloud cover.** Clouds usually put at least some sort of a damper on UVA rays, but they don't filter out UVB, so it's well within the realm of possibility to burn on an overcast day. In fact, 70% of UV rays penetrate through clouds.
- **A cool breeze**, which not only makes it feel as though you're getting less sun than you really are, but also compounds the drying effects of sunlight by wicking surface moisture off the skin.
- **Clothes and hats made from loosely woven materials.** Shop for summer fashions with an eye toward closely woven fabrics like polyester, rayon, and cotton/poly blends. These do a far better job of blocking out UV rays than more open weaves do, such as gauze, linen, and lightweight cotton knits. In hats, look for wide-brimmed styles made from tightly woven fabric. This rules out straw hats, because the open weave permits way too much UV penetration, as well as baseball-style caps, which, though closely woven, don't shade the face and neck as fully as we'd like them to. The ideal solution? A lined hat with a brim broad enough to shade your neck, ears, and face completely.
- **White or very lightly colored T-shirts or tank tops.** The average, off-the-rack white cotton T-shirt provides an SPF of about 5. For that amount of protection, you might as well be nude. The new see-through and sheer blouses aren't any better, and if your shirt gets wet, the SPF approaches zero.

The Straight Dope on Tanning Lamps

The idea that indoor tanning lamps somehow produce a "safe" tan because they don't burn the skin is an incredibly dangerous myth (or scam, take your pick!) that many otherwise intelligent people still believe to be true. But don't you believe it—not even for an instant!

Most indoor sunlamps, including those that supposedly do not generate any UVB light, crank out two to three times the UVA radiation of real sunlight, thus producing rays that not only penetrate deeper into the skin but also fail to provide the protective base tan that occurs through natural exposure. Strangely enough, it would probably be better for the patrons of tanning salons and the owners of home tanning beds if these devices *did* emit UVB. The resulting burn, at least, would give them a painful reminder of the damage being done.

A Day at the (Electric) Beach

The light emitted by an indoor sunlamp is so intense that a single 15- to 30-minute session at your friendly, neighborhood tanning salon exposes you to approximately the same amount of UV radiation you'd experience in a *full day* at the beach. Not surprisingly, recent studies have demonstrated that irregular moles and melanoma—the deadliest form of skin cancer—are much more common in women who frequent tanning salons than in the population as a whole. What a great way to speed up the aging process! Go often enough, and you could look 60 before you reach 40.

THE BARE NECESSITIES: SUNSCREENS, SUNBLOCKS, SELF-TANNERS

Below:

Smile if you're wearing sunscreen!

If you've read this far, you realize that we simply cannot, in good conscience, recommend sunbathing or purposeful tanning of any sort. Nor should we. As skin care experts, we have a professional obligation to give you the straight scoop, which is: NOTHING AGES YOUR SKIN, OR ERODES ITS HEALTH, AS RAPIDLY AND DRAMATICALLY AS UV EXPOSURE.

This being the case, proper sun protection is the only practical option for anyone who wishes to spend quality time outdoors. Now, we

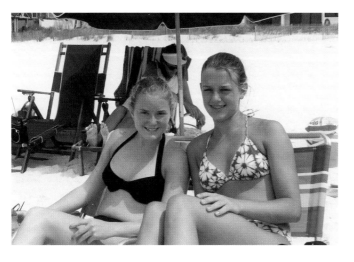

don't expect you to hole up in the basement for the summer, or to clothe yourself from head to toe every time you go out to mow the lawn or meet your friends at the pool. But when you do expose your skin to sunlight for any extended period—and by extended, we mean 15 minutes or longer—it's absolutely vital that you take advantage of the excellent protection offered by the modern sun care products we'll discuss in the remainder of this chapter.

SPF: How Much Is Enough?

To shop the sun care aisle intelligently, you should know a few basic facts about the almost universal, but not always well understood, SPF rating system that manufacturers display on the labels of sunscreens and sunblocks. The acronym "SPF" stands for Sun Protection Factor, a measurement used to rate the UVB filtering or blocking power of products designed to protect skin from solar radiation. You'll notice that we mentioned UVB just now, and *not UVA*. That's because the SPF number alone doesn't give you a clue as to whether a specific product provides UVA protection. For that information, you have to do a little digging, as we'll explain momentarily.

In theory, the SPF rating also tells you how long you can withstand direct UV exposure before burning. The formula supposedly works like this: If you typically burn after 30 minutes of unprotected exposure, an SPF 15 product should allow you to stay outdoors fifteen times longer than normal, in this instance, 7.5 hours (or .5 hour $\times$ 15). Similarly, if you generally burn after 15 minutes outside, an SPF 20 product should keep you untoasted for about 5 hours (or .25 $\times$ 20). Again, that's the theory. But in real life, you shouldn't expect any sunscreen or sunblock, no matter what the SPF, to perform at maximum effectiveness for more than a couple of hours, particularly if you're involved in water sports or in activities that make you sweat.

The SPF rating does, however, provide a meaningful way to compare the protective power of any two products you're thinking of buying: a lower SPF means less protection; a higher SPF, more. So how much protection is adequate? Until very recently, the standard answer has always been SPF 15. Many authorities still stick to that standard, but more and more experts (including us) now advise that you look for an SPF of 30 or higher.

Hmmm . . . Sunscreen? Or Sunblock? Or Does It Even Matter?

There are very real differences between products designed to *block* UV radiation and those designed to *screen* it. Manufacturers, however, have confused the issue no end by using the terms "sunscreen" and "sunblock" as if the two were interchangeable. Sunscreen makers have been the worst offenders, often identifying any broad-spectrum, high SPF product as a sunblock, regardless of whether it truly blocks UV radiation or not. This confusion makes it even more critical than ordinary for you to be an informed consumer: To choose wisely, you'll need to know how screens and blocks differ, and how to recognize one from the other, by reading the label and list of ingredients correctly.

Sunscreens

Sunscreens, in the true sense of the term, are sun care products that chemically absorb and filter UV rays to protect your skin. Since the rays are not blocked out entirely, some UV penetration does take place. Most sunscreens, and nearly all high-SPF varieties, are extremely effective at filtering UVB light and thus preventing burns. On the UVA side, though, the results vary widely—from no protection whatsoever, to partial protection, to nearly complete protection. So what do you look for? Three things, mainly:

1. **Broad-spectrum protection**, which indicates that the product filters UVA rays as well as UVB. Most brands will promote the fact that their product offers both types of protection, but if you're in doubt, just check the list of active ingredients. The presence of *avobenzone*, *titanium*, or *zinc oxide* on that list means that UVA rays will be filtered to a fairly high degree.

2. **A hypoallergenic formula**, which reduces the odds that you'll suffer an allergic reaction when you apply the product to your skin or wear it on a sunny day. The first type of reaction is called *allergic contact dermatitis*; the second, a *photosensitive reaction*.[6] Though a number of common sunscreen ingredients

are potentially allergenic, *benzophenones*, *cinnamates*, and *PABA* (short for para-aminobenzoic acid) seem to account for most of the damage. Watch out, too, for PABA derivatives, such as *padimate-O* and *padimate-A*, if you find that you're sensitive to PABA. Finally, avobenzone is also known to induce allergic reactions in some people, but with much less frequency than the other ingredients we've mentioned.

3. Some degree of water or sweat resistance. According to FDA guidelines, a sunscreen or sunblock must maintain full effectiveness under water for 80 minutes in order to be labeled "waterproof." For products identified as "water resistant," the standard drops to half that time, or 40 minutes. You should keep this in mind if you swim, exercise, sail, surf, or water ski with any regularity. Very few of us, after all, head to the lake or the seashore for a quick, half-hour visit. We usually make a day of it. Our rule of thumb is that sun protection ought to be reapplied each and every time you come out of the water. Friction from waves, water temperature, the wind, and towel-drying all erode protection faster than you think. And when you reapply, don't be stingy. It takes a full ounce—enough to fill a shot glass or the palm of your hand—for a sunscreen or sunblock to cover you completely and still live up to its SPF rating. So if you err, err on the side of overgenerosity. This is one instance in which what seems like too much is probably not enough!

Water Skiers: Treat Your Feet to a Burn-Free Tow!
Water skiers, as well as surfers and jet skiers, need to be especially attentive to their feet. Sun protection gets stripped off at warp speed as you zip through the water, subjecting the tender skin of the arches and toes to potentially nasty burns. After a day of unprotected skiing—or hanging ten—it's not uncommon for the feet to burn and swell so badly that just *trying* to put on shoes and socks brings excruciating pain.

We have a friend, as a matter of fact, whose size-14 feet were once burned to the point that they looked like two gigantic

Below:
Don't forget to apply sunscreen to all exposed areas whenever you're wearing skin-baring styles!

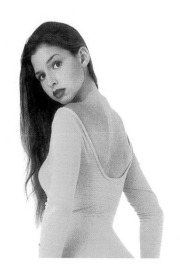

boiled lobsters less than an hour after he'd finished water skiing. Diners in a lakeside restaurant later noticed those burns from a good quarter mile away, and were gesturing and pointing from their window seats as he disembarked the boat and gingerly walked toward them, shoes in hand. Suffice to say, he did not enjoy himself much that evening, or for several days after!

The solution: Use the waxiest, ultra-high SPF sunblock (or sunscreen) you can find, and reapply it religiously throughout the day. Some of the new varieties designed for sports usage, such as Coppertone Sport SPF 48, Banana Boat Maximum Block SPF 50, Beaver 43, and Extreme, offer the heavy-duty protection, water resistance, and staying power you want.

Hot Spots!

It's a fact: You can use a boatload of SPF 30 sunblock and still burn if you're not thorough about covering yourself *everywhere*. Most people who miss spots seem to miss them in the following areas, which we call the "hot spots."

- ears
- back
- nose
- hair part
- along the hairline (don't want to mess up that 'do!)

Remember, too, that since basal cell carcinoma accounts for 80% of new skin cancer cases, you do yourself a real service by applying heavy coverage to the places where it starts—namely, the head, neck, and hands.

Lip Service

When you put on sunscreen, it's easy to forget your lips. But the sun won't miss them! To keep yours from becoming dry, cracked, and blistered, use a sunscreen or UV filtering balm specifically designed for the lips. Clinique, Chapstick, and Neutrogena, among others, offer lip screens that do an admirable job of providing both the UV protection and moisture you need. Make a habit of carrying a stick in your purse— and use it often!

Eye Wear & Sun Care

Sunglasses are the one form of sun protection that most folks don't quibble with a whole lot. Few people, we suppose, really want to squint all day, and there are more than enough styles available to suit just about everyone's taste. When you buy your next pair, look for polarized shades (darker is better) that offer both UVA and UVB protection. Also, choose glasses with lenses sufficiently large to fully protect the sensitive areas surrounding your eyes. The dreaded "crow's feet" you see encircling the eyes of so many older women are a direct result of (three guesses?) too much UV exposure.

Sunblocks

In contrast to sunscreens, products accurately labeled as sunblocks do not filter sunlight; they literally form a protective barrier between your skin and UV radiation. Sunblocks can be divided into two types, both of which offer outstanding broad-spectrum protection:

- traditional, chemical-based blocks
- newer, non-chemical blocks

Chemical-based sunblocks prevent UV penetration through their opacity, which reflects and scatters the sun's rays when they bombard the surface of your skin. In practice, this means that the more protection you want, the more of the stuff you have to smear on, since a thicker coat results in greater opacity. Until just a few years ago, these products tended to be thick, oily pastes like zinc oxide ointment, which was a favorite of the serious beach-going crowd. Problem was, they were greasy, stained clothes, and left behind a milky film after application. Many of our readers, no doubt, are old enough to have seen a lifeguard or two soaking up the sun with a streak of shiny white goo running the length of his nose. Those were the older blocks—terrific as solar protection, but not much to look at, and a real mess to apply.

The newer blocks, which were pioneered by Neutrogena in the early 1990s, pair an almost transparent form of zinc oxide with finely ground titanium dioxide particles to create a *physical* barrier between your skin and UV radiation. These products, in our estimation, possess some distinct advantages over both sunscreens and traditional sunblocks:

- Since they are "non-chemical formulas," allergic reactions to them are relatively rare.
- They go on clear, and are generally easier to apply than chemical-based blocks.
- They offer broad-spectrum protection that is as good as—and often better than—the protection offered by chemical-based products with the same SPF.

Two to try: SkinMedica Daily Sun Protection with daily anti-aging formula and SkinCentials Daily Sun Defense SPF 20. For those who prefer a block with a dry, powder-matte finish, SkinMedica also offers Safesun Dry Finish Daily Anti-Aging Formula.

Put It On . . .

Like the soaps we discussed in Chapter Two, sunscreens must chemically bind with the skin to be effective. Consequently, you'll want to apply them indoors at least 30 minutes before you go out, to give the product time to establish itself on the skin's surface. Non-chemical sunblocks, conversely, can be applied just before you go out the door, though it's still a good idea to put them on inside before you begin to perspire. Try different screens or blocks until you find one that feels good on your skin. Higher SPFs, as we've noted, afford greater protection, despite the widespread belief that SPF 15 is all you need. Again, to our way of thinking, you want SPF 30 or higher. In fact, the higher the better.

Unless you have very oily skin, avoid alcohol-based gel blocks. They disappear on the skin, and it's hard to know if you've missed a spot. If you use a gel, apply it in a systematic fashion to ensure that you cover every part of your body. First coat your legs, then your front, then the back, then the arms, and finally the face.[7] In addition, most alcohol-based gels can take off nail polish (a scary thought!), so be careful around your hands.

To apply sunscreen on your back, use an applicator with a long handle (available in most surgical supply stores, or make your own by wrapping a washcloth around the end of a back scratcher). Spray-on sunblocks are another good option for hard-to-reach areas. Neutrogena makes an oil-free, waterproof spray we like especially well: It's rub-resistant, sweat-resistant, and doesn't feel heavy on the skin the way some oilier products do. Plus, it produces a fine, even mist that makes it mercifully easy and quick to apply.

And Keep Putting It On . . .

Always remember that a sunscreen can only protect you for a limited amount of time, which varies depending on the product's SPF, its greasiness, and the thickness of the coat you apply. However, even the best sunscreen, liberally applied, won't last forever. Get into the habit of keeping sun protection in your purse, backpack, or beach bag; then reapply it at regular intervals whenever you're out for more than a couple of hours. You'll want to determine a reasonable length of time between applications (2 hours or less is a good starting point), watch the clock, and stick to your plan. Like most good habits, this will be a bit of a pain at first, but will become second nature after just a few repetitions. The reward, of course, is that your chances of burning now—and of suffering serious skin damage later in life—will be drastically reduced. Not a bad trade-off, if you ask us.

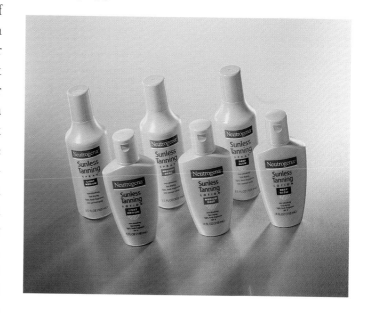

Above:
The only safe way to "sunbathe" is indoors with a self-tanner.

A TOTALLY TUBULAR TAN: THE ONLY SAFE ALTERNATIVE

If there were an award for "most improved cosmetic product," it would have to go to self-tanners. Back when self-tanners were initially introduced, many of them gave the skin an unnaturally orange cast, smelled funny, and were prone to dissolve and streak at the first sign of moisture. Today's products, however, are good enough to make you wonder, health concerns aside, why some people still bother with a sun-induced tan. The best self-tanners nowadays are completely odor-free, relatively easy to apply, and, most important, offer a convincing, natural-looking tan without the dangers of UV exposure.

Self-tanners, whether they are packaged as lotions, creams, powders, gels, or sprays, come in two basic varieties: bronzers and skin stains. While neither variety is head over heels better than the other, there are unique advantages and drawbacks to each. As you'll see, the crucial question is: Do you prefer a product that's easy to wash off? Or one that stays on longer after you apply it?

For those of us who want a dash of color every now and then, but don't care to live with it for several days, bronzers are the appropriate option. A bronzer, in most instances, is a suntan-colored makeup, similar in composition and effect to color-correcting creams in other shades such as white and green. Most bronzers utilize a water-soluble pigment to make your skin appear tanned. Because the pigment is water-soluble, bronzers are typically very easy to remove: You simply wash them off with soap and warm water, just as you would other types of makeup. That's the plus side, especially if you're not happy with your initial attempt to apply the stuff and wish to start over. The downside with bronzers is that they don't last too long, and so require constant reapplication if you get the look you want and wish to maintain it.

Skin stains, on the other hand, are the right choice for people who want an artificial tan that offers greater staying power and requires less maintenance. Of course, you will never see these products identified as "stains" by the manufacturer. Usually, a more appealing name like "tanning mist" or "self-tanning lotion" is used on the label. To add to the confusion, many are even called bronzers. (But just get some on a white blouse, and you'll realize soon enough that they are, indeed, stains!) Self-tanners that darken your skin through staining contain a dye called DHA, or dihydroxyacetone. DHA chemically binds with the cells on your skin's surface to darken them and create a tanned color. The depth of color produced by a given tanner varies according to the amount of DHA it contains, typically somewhere between 2 and 5 percent, depend-

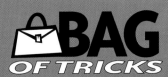

How To Apply Self-Tanning Products

Step 1: The Body

The best way to apply a self-tanner to your body is to first remove dead skin cells with a loofah sponge. In principle, what you're doing here equates to what a house painter does when he scrapes and scrubs the walls down before painting them: You're priming the surface of your skin for a smooth, even coat of coloring. For the same reason, you should also shave your legs. But do not moisturize afterward, since the water in your moisturizer can serve to dilute the tanner.

Now, you're just about ready to apply a nice, even coat of the tanning product according to the manufacturer's directions. But to play it safe, you should at this point test the product on a small, hidden patch of skin to be sure that you like the shade, and also to get a sense of how many coats it will take to achieve the desired look. Go lightly to start, then layer on additional coats until the test area has attained the depth of color you're after. Exercising patience and using a light touch are important when applying self-tanners, because you can always add more lotion to deepen the shade if the coat is insufficient. But if you overstain,

it's really difficult and time-consuming to get back to your natural skin color. But more on that later.

Once you're satisfied that the test area looks correct, go ahead and start spreading on the tanner. Do so as evenly as possible over all the areas you wish to appear tanned, and rub the product in vigorously. Begin with the feet to avoid getting crease marks across your stomach when bending to reach the lower body, then work your way up. Try not to miss spots, and do not try to economize. To prevent dark patches, rub gently around rough areas like the ankles, knees, and elbows, where tanner tends to collect.

When you reach the top of the thighs, you can either stop there and skip the pelvis, to create a "bathing suit" tan, or simply continue coating from thighs to pelvis to stomach. As you work your way up the torso, fade the tan up to—or onto—your breasts, according to your preference. If you use a different brand of tanner for your face than for your body, rub the facial product down to your neck, upper chest, and breasts to ensure an exact match and consistent coloring.

Step 2: The Face

Use the same tanner on your face as you do on your body, unless your tanner of choice comes with a specific face-only component, then proceed as follows:

1. Wash, exfoliate gently, use a toner to remove superficial oil, and then rinse. If you have a dry complexion, however, you can probably get by with simply washing and rinsing. Allow your skin to dry completely, and *do not* apply moisturizer.

2. Start applying tanner at your forehead, being careful to avoid your eyebrows and the fine hairs along your hairline (that is, unless you wish to dye them, too!).

3. Do not apply DHA-based tanner to the sensitive skin within the oval-shaped area defined by your eye socket. Your eyes will really smart if you get tanner in them, and it's easier and cleaner to use a powder or gel bronzer to blend the tan up to your eyes.

4. Avoiding your lips, bring tanner down over your ears, chin, neck, and onto your chest, as we described earlier.

Step 3: The Hands

As odd as it may sound, applying tanner to your hands can be the trickiest part of the whole process. First, make sure that you've completely covered your face and body with tanner and that the product has been thoroughly rubbed in everywhere. If that's the case, wash your hands well. Once your hands are dry, squirt a dab of self-tanner onto the back of one hand, then rub the backs of your hands together, blending down toward the forearms. Admittedly, it's awkward to work this way, but you don't want tanner on your palms if you can help it. Be careful, too, around your cuticles and nails; they'll absorb tanner, and typically turn a very unappealing shade of orange or yellow if stained.

Step 4: Problem Areas

Even if you're extremely careful during application, tanner still wants to collect on the rough skin covering your elbows, kneecaps, ankle bones, and Achilles tendons, resulting in a comparatively darker look in these areas. To lighten them up for a good match, simply wet a piece of tissue, and swab gently until you reach the correct shade. This same trick can also be used for lightening the inner part of your arm between the wrist and elbow. Since this area tends to be less tanned under natural circumstances, you'll have a more realistic looking effect if you lighten it a tad.

Step 5: Drying & Touch-Up

Self-tanners usually take from 15 to 30 minutes to dry to the point that they won't stain clothing or furniture. Read the package to find the specific drying time for the product you use. As to what to do while the stuff dries, there are basically two options: One, walk around nude and don't touch a thing; and two, find an old black or dark-colored T-shirt in your closet and some shorts to match, then go about your business. The second option is obviously more convenient, and most self-tanning products can be effectively laundered from dark fabrics. Of course, no matter which route you take, you'll want to wait until the product has completely dried before changing into nicer clothes.

If, after the product has dried, you notice a few mistakes, fill in any spots that are too pale with an additional (light!) coat of tanner, and remove excess tanner from places that are too dark. For spots that are too dark, remove dried tanner by scrubbing hard with a damp washcloth. If you remove too much, just add more later. But don't, for heaven's sake, use anything harsher than soap and water to take off that first coat.

ing on the formula. Obviously, the more DHA, the darker the shade.

Artificial tans produced by DHA-based products generally last 3 or 4 days, or about the time it takes your epidermis to slough off all of the cells you originally stained. That being the case, these products simplify your life by making maintenance far less of a chore, but can present problems if you're not satisfied with the color that results. Apply too much—or choose a product in a shade you don't care for—and you're essentially stuck with the look for half a week or so.

PRODUCT SPOTLIGHT   Self Tanners

Before we give you specific product recommendations, a word of warning: The great majority of self-tanner packages are inadequately labeled. We've already mentioned the confusion caused by manufacturers who don't distinguish between bronzers that contain DHA (stains) and those that don't (color-correcting creams). To make matters even more perplexing, tanners come in an array of formulations for different complexions and skin types. The best advice, especially if you are at all fair complected, is to begin with a package marked "for pale skin," "fair," "light," or the equivalent. If the coloring isn't deep enough to suit you, you can easily add a second coat or switch to a darker shade the next day. But if you start too dark, you live with the look—or sentence yourself to an awful lot of vigorous scrubbing that may or may not succeed in returning your skin to its natural shade. As we've said before, it's far better to start light and then darken by degrees than to attempt the reverse.

Our Recommended List

For the face: Estee Lauder, Clarins, and Clinique offer some wonderful lotions. For sensitive or acne-prone skin, Lancome's formula won't cause breakouts.

For the body: La Prairie's mouse moisturizers; Clarins gel (dries in minutes); Bovannah (with built-in sunscreen); Christian Dior or Clinique lotions, both of which come in color-coded packages to indicate depth of shading.

Try also: Estee Lauder Self-Action Sunless Super Tan, a new line of self-tanning solutions that turn your skin a deeper, more natural tan color. They dry fast, tan fast, and (bingo!) don't streak. Available in easy-on lotions and sprays.

Well worth a shot: Neutrogena Sunless Tanning Spray Deep Glow offers such a nice, natural-looking tan that you can almost forgive the incredibly long name. Dries fast without streaks, and the one-touch continuous spray helps you cover those hard-to-reach places.

Self Tanners *Are Not* Sunscreens

Don't be fooled into thinking you have a protective base tan just because a self-tanner makes your skin appear darker! Fact is, most self-tanners are strictly cosmetic products; they do not stimulate melanin production in the manner of a natural, sun-induced tan; nor do they filter or block UV rays in the manner of a sunscreen. So unless the package specifically states that your self-tanner contains sunscreen (and some brands do), you still need to take precautions.

Just Your Type . . .

As with soaps and cosmetics, it's important to match your sun care protection to your skin type. A few simple guidelines should get you pointed in the right direction:

- *For normal to dry skin*—avoid oil-free products, since they often contain alcohol or glycerin, which can be excessively drying to your skin, especially if you're outdoors and already losing moisture to the sun and wind. Instead, opt for oil-based products or water-based products that contain moisturizing oils or emollients.
- *For oily skin*—oil-free formulas are best. But if your complexion is only moderately oily, a water-based product with some oil content may work well, too.
- *For acne-prone or problem skin*—oil-free is a must, but excessive drying can be an issue too, so look for water-based products designed specifically for sensitive skin.

WHEN DRIVING, PLEASE . . .

Don't dangle your arm out the driver's side window. It looks hokey, and you'd be amazed at the number of people who suffer sun damage on the back of their left forearm and hand but nowhere else. So roll that bad boy up: Glass does a marvelous job of blocking most UV rays, and you can always use the passenger window for ventilation or a little fresh air.

YOU CAN BE UNTANNED . . . AND STILL LOOK HOT!

The hottest looking women on the beach or at the pool aren't necessarily the most tanned ones. More often, in fact, they're the ones with toned muscles, a tight tummy, the right makeup, and fashions that bring out their best features to the max. All of which, of course, requires more work and forethought than lounging in the sun for hours on end.

Why not prove to yourself that you don't need to tan to turn heads this summer? If you're fit, you can show some skin with-

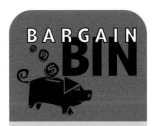

BARGAIN BIN

Banana Tanna!

One of our favorite self-tanners, Banana Boat Sunless Tanning Spray, is both inexpensive and available at nearly any drugstore. It's most intriguing feature is that you can adjust the color to your liking. Light, medium, and dark are all in one bottle. Plus, the more often you use it, the deeper your artificial tan becomes.

out a tan—and we promise, nobody important will mind one bit. If you want your skin to appear a tad darker than it really is, use warm makeup shades and bronzers, add highlights to your hair, or try a toothpaste specially formulated for whitening. For an attention-getting look, wear bright, vibrant clothes, or choose a swimsuit in an eye-catching color like jet black, copper, or silver metallic.

Believe us now: In the summertime, suntanned women are as plentiful as ants at a picnic. But a woman with a signature style is much harder to find. If you haven't already begun to develop yours, start now, and we suspect you'll get noticed plenty—in the summer and all year round.

END NOTES

1. This is just one more reason to worry about that giant hole in the ozone, which researchers have estimated to be as large as continental Europe at times, and which periodically appears and disappears over the polar ice caps. Though scientists continue to debate whether global warming poses an *immediate* threat to human health, we hope that today's young people will do more than previous generations have done to protect and preserve the atmosphere that makes life on this planet possible. The fact that ancient glaciers are gradually melting in places as far removed as the Swiss Alps and Western Antarctica suggests that we may have less time to solve the problem than we'd like to think.

2. Strong evidence exists, too, that extensive UV exposure suppresses the immune system and thus reduces our capacity to ward off illnesses of all kinds. This is why you are more likely to become ill *after returning* from a warm-weather vacation than *during* your stay in Hawaii or Florida.

3. To find striking examples of the fashions of the time, just check out an art history book with famous late 19th-century paintings in it. The aristocratic women portrayed by masters like Cézanne, Matisse, and Sargent are virtually always clothed from head to toe when shown in outdoor settings.

4. The bikini, you might be surprised to learn, was invented shortly after World War II, in 1947!

5. For many years, cartoonist Gerry Trudeau's classic comic strip *Doonesbury* featured a character named Zonker Harris. Zonker's principal ambition in life was to achieve the perfect tan, and he pursued it religiously in strip after strip during the 1970s and 80s. Folks in our generation found this funny, of course, because most of us knew someone not too unlike Trudeau's fictional sun-worshipper. The artist himself, however, ultimately came down with skin cancer, and subsequently created a series of strips that showed a reformed Zonker using sunscreen and retiring from the sunbathing scene.

6. Chemicals or substances that trigger allergic reactions on skin that has been exposed to sunlight are known as *photosensitizers*, and they are by no means restricted to sun care products only. They can also be found in many cosmetics, deodorants, over-the-counter medications, and even in certain foods. It's worth noting that food-related reactions typically result from handling, not eating, the photosensitizing item, so you're more likely to encounter them as a cook than as a diner.

7. Even if you don't use a gel, developing a consistent system for sunscreen application is a good idea. You'll be much less likely to miss spots, and you'll probably put the stuff on faster and more efficiently by virtue of having a routine.

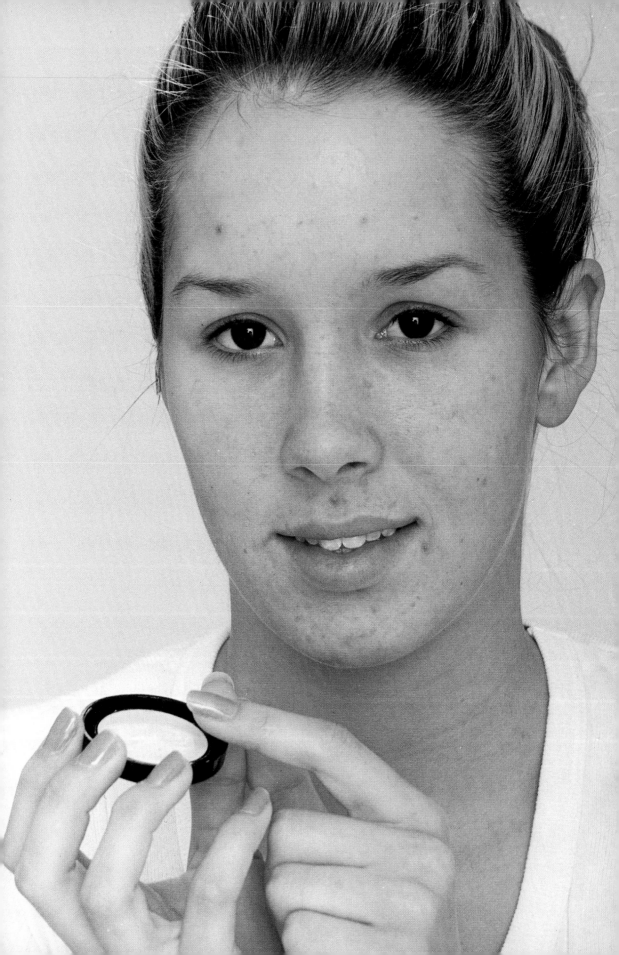

That Three-Letter Word, *Zit:* Need We Say More?

We have chosen to use the slang term *zit* when speaking of pimples in a general sense. Why? Because *zit*, in three short angry letters, so accurately conveys the true terror of what faces you in the bathroom mirror the moment you spot one. Zits, as we all know, are rude little critters. They possess a sixth sense that enables them to erupt, as if by magic, on the most crucial days of our lives. When, after all, was the last time you heard a story about a zit that *disappeared* the day before the prom or the morning of a big job interview?

Among other useful tidbits, you will discover in the following pages that the impeccably horrendous timing of your breakouts is probably not the result of rotten luck or evil spirits, but an outcome of emotional stress and the increased hormonal activity it produces. But before we delve too deeply into the causes of acne, we must first learn more about the disease itself, and the different kinds of zits it produces.

TYPES OF ACNE

Experts in dermatology have identified three major types of acne:

- *acne vulgaris*, which is also called "teen" acne, although adults occasionally suffer from it, too
- *acne rosacea*, which is commonly referred to as "adult" acne, because it primarily afflicts people between the ages of 20 and 50 (and can develop into a chronic, lifelong condition)
- *perioral dermatitis*, which causes clusters of pimples to form around the "muzzle" of the face (i.e., the sides of the nose, the skin around the mouth, and the chin)

In this chapter, we will concern ourselves chiefly, but not exclusively, with acne vulgaris, because it accounts for the overwhelming majority of the acne problems experienced by teens. A quick glance around your classroom, workplace, or maybe even your family dinner table will demonstrate that "teen" acne manifests itself differently from person to person and from outbreak to outbreak. The most visible evidence of the disease, obviously, is our good friend, the zit.

The Definitive . . . Zit!

So, just what is a zit? Well, according to *Stedman's Medical Dictionary*, a zit (or pimple, to use the dictionary's term) can be defined as "a papule or small pustule; usually meant to denote a lesion of acne." Translated into everyday language, this means that zits are small, typically bump-like eruptions of the skin. They originate in hair follicles (= oil pores) that have become plugged up with a mixture of dead skin cells, bacterial by-products, perspiration, and sebum, the skin's natural lubricant. As you'll recall from Chapter One, sebum is a somewhat thick, greasy fluid produced by the oil (or sebaceous) glands to provide necessary moisture to the epidermis, or outer layer of skin. Ideally, sebum travels slowly and smoothly through a short duct that leads from the oil glands in the dermis to the oil pores on the skin's surface, where it is discharged and gradually dissipates through evaporation, friction, or cleansing.

Birth of a Zit

Zits crop up when the body produces too much sebum to be efficiently discharged through the pores. When this occurs, the sebum—which is gooey stuff to begin with—starts to accumulate somewhere either below or near the opening of the follicle, where it mingles with debris, thickens, and eventually hardens. At the same time, the cells that compose the walls of the oil duct also tend to thicken, which further restricts the free, natural flow of oil.

The resulting blockage causes the skin immediately surrounding the plugged follicle to fill to the bulging point with oily, bacteria-laden fluid. In time, the entire area becomes inflamed, which is a nice way of saying that it swells, reddens, and generally looks just awful. Excess sebum accounts for the swelling around the head of a zit, while the infection caused by bacterial waste products accounts for the red, angry color of the bump.

These waste products, incidentally, are fatty acids produced by the legions of bacteria that live along the walls of your oil ducts, happily feeding on the sebum and nutrients that pass their way. Under normal circumstances, such bacteria pose no problems to your skin. But as sebum production increases and oil builds up beneath the skin surrounding a clogged pore, two ugly events take place: first, the bacterial population grows rapidly, owing to the more plentiful food supply, and therefore generates greater quantities of fatty acid waste; and second, that waste, now released from the confines of the oil duct, irritates and inflames the surrounding skin it comes in contact with. In short, a zit has been born—perhaps with you (or one of us!) as the proud parent.

Name That Zit: Papules, Pustules, Whiteheads, Blackheads, & Cysts

Of course, not all zits are created equal. In fact, they differ widely in terms of size, appearance, and severity. Some appear as large, nearly bruise-sized welts; others show up as the tiniest of red bumps. Some are extremely tender and painful to the touch; others cause little or no physical discomfort. Some can be treated with special cleansers and common topical ointments available in any drugstore; others may require stronger prescribed medications or surgical removal by a dermatologist. But all zits, as we have seen, stem from blockage of the skin's oil ducts. Two principal factors determine what type of zit results from a specific blockage: where the blockage occurs within the duct, and whether the opening of the affected pore is open or closed.

A blockage that occurs at or very near the surface of the skin typically produces one of four types of zits:

- *papules*, which are small, inflamed (= red) zits lacking the familiar "head" that characterizes whiteheads and pustules
- *pustules*, also lovingly referred to as pus-heads, which are larger red bumps capped by a festive crown of whitish pus protruding from the opening of the pore
- *whiteheads*, which resemble pustules in some respects, except that the pus-head is completely enclosed under the opening of the pore and the surrounding skin is not inflamed
- *blackheads*, which display a dark (some would say dirty looking) head and no inflammation of the surrounding skin

Much of the difference between pustules, whiteheads, and blackheads can be attributed to the size of the opening of the affected oil pore: If the opening has contracted to the extent that fluid cannot easily escape, the result is a pustule or whitehead. In pustules, the pore, though constricted, remains open; in whiteheads, it is closed. If the pore's opening is somewhat larger, a *blackhead* typically results. With blackheads, you won't see the surrounding redness of a papule or pustule, nor much of a bump, if any at all, because the problem area is almost entirely confined to the pore itself. Also, it's worth noting that blackheads don't derive their dark coloring from dirt or grime on the surface of your skin, but from pigment that has latched on to the oily fluid during its journey from the sebaceous gland to the oil pore.

Zits that form as a result of deep, subsurface blockages often create *cysts*. In this type of zit, sebum accumulates far enough below the skin's surface that the fluid has no opportunity to drain, which eventually causes the swollen oil gland to rupture. In time, a sac forms around the site of the rupture and becomes filled with a gummy, off-white substance composed of dead skin cells and the contents of the damaged gland. The deeply embedded bumps that ensue are usually larger, more tender, and more difficult to treat than any of the other kinds of zits we've discussed thus far. The sac containing the cyst, in particular, can prove especially resistant to treatment. It tends to cling tightly to neighboring tissue, and will often reappear even after a cyst has been lanced or surgically removed. If even a miniscule portion of the sac remains after treatment, the potential exists for the formation of a new cyst at the site of the old one. Last, some cysts will ooze a clear, almost watery fluid to the skin's surface and present a red, inflamed appearance; others will be dry to the touch and possess the surface coloring of normal skin.

Since cysts can appear alone or as part of acne, it's not at all uncommon for an individual to get the odd cyst every now and again. In some instances, an individual cyst will heal on its own; in others, a dermatologist's care will be required to treat or remove it. But when cysts appear in bunches, this indicates a very severe form of acne (called cystic acne) that *necessitates* professional attention. While there are many things you can do at home to cope with minor outbreaks of small papules, pustules, whiteheads, or blackheads, trying to handle cystic acne without qualified help can easily lead to permanent scarring and rapid worsening of the condition. Don't make that mistake! See your dermatologist right away if your acne bumps seem deeply embedded, overly large, or especially painful.

Perioral Dermatitis: A Real Mouthful

If you notice clusters of small, tightly clumped zits around the sides of your mouth, along the sides of your nose and on your chin, you may have a condition known as perioral dermatitis.

Unlike most types of acne, which tend to hit males harder than females, this one typically affects women. The current consensus among medical professionals is that perioral dermatitis can be brought on by prolonged use of many common food and drug products, including:

- corticosteroid creams
- tartar-control toothpastes
- scented cosmetics
- chewing gum, especially cinnamon flavored varieties

Though we don't know precisely why these products seem to induce zits, we do know that it takes several years of repeated use for the condition to develop. Patients are therefore often surprised when the offending item is identified, and respond by saying, "No way. I've been using that since I was a kid!" And in many cases, the specific product cannot be determined with certainty. Even so, several effective treatments exist. Oral antibiotics like tetracycline and minocycline have enjoyed good success rates, as have topical medications that contain sulfur and salicylic acid as active ingredients. Depending on the severity of the case, a doctor may prescribe one of the oral or topical drugs on its own, or use one of each type in combination. For most patients, improvement begins to show after two to eight weeks of treatment.

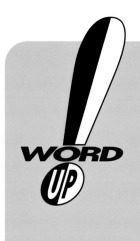

WORD UP

The technical term *comedo* is used to describe a single white-head or blackhead; its plural form is *comedones*. A whitehead is referred to as a *closed comedo*, a blackhead as an *open comedo*. Of course, we don't expect you to fling these terms around in ordinary conversation, unless you wish to impress (or perhaps annoy) your friends. But they are handy to know when you shop for cosmetics and other skin care products. Products or ingredients that are known to cause whiteheads or blackheads are said to be *comedogenic*; those that are known not to cause them are defined as a *non-comedogenic*. For obvious reasons, you will never run across a product label identifying an item as comedogenic, but you will find several in nearly every skin care category labeled as non-comedogenic. All else being equal, these are smart choices for breakout-prone skin.

GRADES OF ACNE

Many skin care professionals use a grading system to distinguish between mild, moderate, and more severe cases of acne. This system is, of necessity, built on very general guidelines, so you may find it difficult, just looking in the mirror, to decide what grade of acne you have. But if you've read carefully about the various types of acne bumps, you should get a good idea of where you stand within the mild to severe spectrum. Personally, we feel that any grade of acne ought to be looked at by a dermatologist, if for no other reason than to offer reassurance that your problems are minimal. That said, acne is graded according to the following scale:

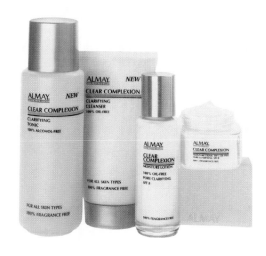

Above:
A variety of affordable, effective cleansing products are designed for correcting oily, acne-prone skin.

Grade 1

This is the mildest type of outbreak, consisting solely of comedones, or non-inflamed whiteheads and blackheads. Grade 1 acne usually won't require any sort of special treatment beyond sensible cleansing and occasional use of mild over-the-counter acne remedies. If, however, you haven't had any luck with the benzoyl peroxide ointments that dominate drugstore shelves, a therapeutic after-cleansing product is often a good alternative for self-treatment. Try SkinMedica Acne Toner, which contains alpha-hydroxy acid and salicylic acid, to eliminate blackheads and tighten pores, or Triaz 6% cleanser from Medicis (requires a prescription).

Grade 2

Grade 2 outbreaks represent moderate acne of the kind experienced by most teenagers. These typically consist of whiteheads and blackheads, as above, as well as small, minimally inflamed papules and pustules. While uncomfortable, most grade 2 outbreaks do not result in permanent scarring or pockmarks.

Grade 3

Acne at this level is regarded as severe, with the skin exhibiting not only whiteheads and blackheads but also deep, inflamed papules and pustules as well. Unlike more moderate outbreaks, grade 3 acne is not confined to the face; it strikes the neck, chest, back, and shoulders, too.

Grade 4

Grade 4 acne—the most severe form of outbreak—is technically known as *acne conglobata* or *cystic acne*. It is characterized by deeply embedded cysts and large, widespread pustules that cause permanent scarring. Grade 4 acne can be very painful, and generally afflicts men more often than women. Also, such severe cases tend to develop somewhat later in life than the milder types of acne—usually between the ages of eighteen and thirty.

ACNE ACTIVATORS: THE CAUSES OF BREAKOUTS

By now, you are probably wondering what causes the excessive sebum production that triggers outbreaks of acne. Well, the scientific community would like to know the answer to that question, too, because we haven't yet pinned down the root causes of acne with absolute certainty. Nor have we achieved a foolproof cure for this extraordinarily widespread disorder. But we do know that genetics (i.e., heredity) and hormonal activity play key roles in acne formation, and that other factors such as emotional stress, fever, sore throat, allergies, hives, and allergic reactions to certain skin care products, cosmetics, and medications can aggravate an existing case of acne or give rise to a flare-up.

The Role of Androgens in Acne Formation

A surge in the production of a group of hormones collectively known as *androgens*, in particular, seems directly linked to the development of acne, especially among adolescents and teens. Both men and women secrete androgens, or "male" hormones, so called because they prompt the expression of male sexual characteristics like facial hair growth and the development of large, bulky muscles. Men, however, generally secrete them in greater numbers and are therefore more likely than women to suffer from severe or problem acne.

Many androgens, such as *corticosteroid* and *testosterone*, fall into the steroid family of hormones, and it has been well established that these substances serve to trigger a chain of events that often culminates in acne. The process works like this: High levels of androgen in the bloodstream enlarge the oil glands, which in turn causes a rise in sebum production and thickening of the cells that line the walls of the oil ducts, thus setting the stage for one of the various types of breakouts we described above.

Acne & Your Period

This catalytic (or triggering) effect is usually most pronounced at the onset of puberty and during the teen years, when hormonal activity increases dramatically in both sexes. That's why so many of us experience our worst bouts of acne as teenagers. But you can also observe the process at work among both teen and adult women in connection with the menstrual cycle. Some 60% to 70% of women, in fact, suffer acne breakouts tied to the heightened hormonal levels that occur about a week before their period actually starts. In some cases, these breakouts can be controlled or even eliminated by drugs designed to correct hormonal imbalances. In others, the flare-ups may be so minor and short-lived that your dermatologist will advise that you allow them to subside on their own. But either way, the first step is to take note of when the breakouts happen in relation to your cycle. This will give you—and your dermatologist—a clue to whether the acne is linked to your period.

Pregnancy, Birth Control, & Acne

If you've read much at all about acne, you are probably aware that pregnant women and women who take certain types of birth control pills sometimes experience hormonally induced breakouts. But did you know that pregnancy or ingestion of an oral contraceptive can sometimes help clear up acne as well? Though this might seem contradictory, there are logical reasons that explain why the skin reacts differently under apparently similar circumstances.

Let's start with pregnancy. During the first trimester, an expecting mother undergoes a surge in hormonal activity and therefore produces greater quantities of both female (estrogen) and male (androgen) hormones. If the woman had relatively low levels of male hormones in her system before pregnancy, the increased number of androgens after conception may cause her to break out. On the other hand, if the woman was acne-prone prior to conception, the increased presence of estrogens may help to offset a previously high androgen level and thereby offer her temporary relief from breakouts. The effects of pregnancy on a woman's complexion, then, depend greatly on how it affects her androgen-estrogen balance, which, of course, varies from one individual to the next. For most pregnant women, these changes in the tendency to break out or not break out are temporary, seldom lasting beyond the first three months of the term.

The mixed results experienced by women who take oral contraceptives are also based on hormonal "triggers." Here, the key difference between breaking out and clearing up can be attributed to product ingredients. That's because birth control pills, like the human body, contain both androgen-like and estrogen-like substances to varying degrees.[1] Oral contraceptives that are more heavily weighted toward the androgen side are known as *progesterone-dominant* pills; those that are weighted toward the estrogen side are called *estrogen-dominant* pills. As you might have guessed, progesterone-dominant products are more likely to prompt or worsen acne breakouts, and estrogen-dominant products are more likely to prevent or curtail them. If you are prone to breakouts *and* take birth control pills regularly, we believe it makes good sense to choose a drug that will perform double duty as contraceptive and acne medication. In most cases, your gynecologist should be able to prescribe a product that handles both tasks safely and effectively.

FAMILY MATTERS: ACNE & GENETICS

Severe, deeply embedded acne is often determined by genetics. Not surprisingly, most people who suffer from it have at least one parent who experienced the same problem. Likewise, very stubborn acne commonly plagues those with inherited hormonal conditions such as cystic ovaries and excessive hair growth. With deeply embedded acne, pores get blocked well below the skin's surface, so topical treatments may have a difficult time penetrating effectively enough to reach the site of the plug. In these instances, acne is typically treated with stronger oral medications, usually in tandem with a topical drug of one kind or another. For the very toughest cases, a doctor may prescribe Accutane—a powerful oral medication that we will later describe in more detail.

ACNE: BY THE NUMBERS

Statistics show that acne vulgaris afflicts more than 80% of us at some point during our adolescent years. Remember, too, that acne is not a teens-only condition: Babies get zits. Adults get zits. Pregnant women get zits. In fact, researchers estimate that more than 90% of the general population suffers from one variety of acne or another at least once (and typically, many more times) over the course of their lifetime. So, while we do not wish to minimize the stress, worry, and embarrassment caused by breakouts, acne sufferers can take some consolation in the fact that nearly everyone around them either is, has been, or will be in a similar situation. True, that knowledge probably won't clear up your face for Friday night's dance, but it does suggest that people won't be overly shocked or put off when confronted by a blemished complexion. After all, most of them—including your peers—have been there, done that!

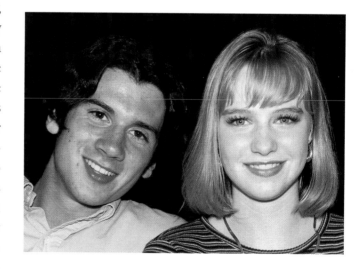

Above:
Keeping acne under control is definitely worth smiling about.

Zit Zones

You've no doubt noticed that zits pop up much more frequently and in greater numbers on the face, back, and chest than elsewhere on the body. The reason? These areas house very dense concentration of oil glands, and so are more susceptible to eruptions of acne.

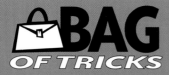

Hiding Acne Bumps

Most makeup experts agree that green is the color of choice for camouflaging zits, since it complements and therefore neutralizes the red coloring of an inflamed acne bump. Some, however, contend that yellow will do the trick in a less obvious and more natural looking manner.[2] Perhaps you should try both and see which works best for you.

To hide a zit, first apply a green (or yellow) tint foundation base to the inflamed area, then cover with your regular makeup. Be careful, though, not to layer on too much foundation or makeup in your effort to conceal the blemish. After all, what you gain by hiding the redness of a zit can easily be negated by unintentionally highlighting its bumpiness.

A helpful tip: If you'd prefer to use a single product as opposed to two when hiding zits, try Lancome's Dual Finish Compact Makeup. It gives you the convenience of a one-step process, plus does a great job of covering red blemishes of all kinds.

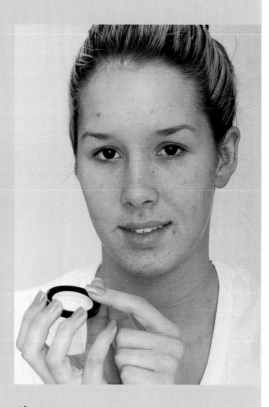

Above:
Corrective concealers in yellow or green are the best choices for hiding acne.

KEEPING ACNE UNDER CONTROL: THE MOST POPULAR OVER-THE-COUNTER DRUGS & PRESCRIBED MEDICATIONS

To date, no one has discovered a definitive cure for acne. But, because the disease affects almost everyone at some time or another, medications designed to treat acne symptoms and prevent future flare-ups constitute big business. Products abound, and change with lightning speed from year to year, and even month to month. Some can be purchased over the counter at your neighborhood drugstore; others must be prescribed by a licensed dermatologist. One word of warning, though: Even the most well known (and, for that reason, seemingly safe) over-the-counter drugs can produce undesirable side effects or be rendered ineffective if you use them incorrectly, as many people unwittingly do.

Consequently, we feel it's always smartest and safest to consult your dermatologist before trying any acne medication. He or she can help you sort through the confusing array of choices that await you in the skin care aisle, make useful suggestions about which products are best for your skin and your type of acne, plus give you sound advice about when to stick with or abandon a medication that doesn't appear to be working. Acne can be an extremely tricky disorder to treat. It appears for a while, then goes into remission, sometime for a few days, sometimes for a month, sometimes for good. What works well for one person, or one kind of acne, may be ineffective for a second, and positively disastrous for a third. By working with your dermatologist from the beginning, chances are that you will not only eliminate much costly and time-consuming trial and error, but also achieve a more effective, lasting solution to your problem.

Fortunately, acne sufferers and their dermatologists have a huge variety of top-flight medications at their disposal. Nearly all of these products, whether sold over the counter or prescribed, attempt to combat acne in one or more of the following ways:

- by removing excess oil from the surface of the skin
- by reducing the bacterial count within the oil ducts
- by controlling hormone levels
- by reducing sebum production

Over-the-counter medications typically focus on fighting bacteria and/or clearing surface oil; prescribed drugs focus on fighting bacteria, controlling hormonal activity, or reducing sebum production. Within both groups, many different forms of medication exist. Some are

Below:
Products for treating acne are all around you—call your dermatologist and check out your drugstore to see what works best for your skin.

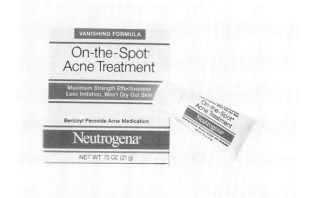

topical agents packaged as cleansers, lotions, and creams; others, almost always prescribed, are taken orally.

As you might expect, the relative strength and potential side effects of any given medication are closely linked: Generally speaking, the more potent the medicine, the more serious the possible side effects. A powerful prescription drug like Accutane, for example, may do wonders to clear up a chronic case of severe acne, but may also cause dryness of the skin, sore muscles, impaired nighttime vision, and other undesirable consequences in patients who use it. By contrast, a relatively mild over-the-counter medication like Oxy-5 or Clearasil probably won't produce any side effects more serious than some superficial dryness, but it may not do much to combat an especially tough case of acne, either.

When selecting acne medications, then, we are almost always in the business of making tradeoffs of one sort or another. To help you better understand the benefits and drawbacks of the many products currently available to acne sufferers, we will examine the key active ingredients used in today's most popular products in a "pros" and "cons" format. Our discussion begins with over-the-counter products, then progresses to prescribed medicines.

Common Ingredients
in Over-the-Counter Drugs

Over-the-counter (or OTC, for short) acne medications use a variety of drying and antibacterial agents as active ingredients. These ingredients, which are meant to dry surface oil and unclog plugged pores, may be used by the manufacturer singly or in combination, and are available in a fairly broad range of strengths. You will find them in products sold as lotions, creams, gels, medicated pads, and cleansers. Nowadays, some are even included in cosmetics. The most widely used of the OTC acne fighters are:

Sulfur & Resorcinol
What: Peeling and antibacterial agents found in many clear and flesh-colored creams and lotions. Often paired with salicylic acid and/or benzoyl peroxide.

Pros: Helps keep your complexion free of excess oil, but doesn't cause undue dryness in most formulations.

Cons: Effectiveness is limited to mild and moderate cases of acne; can be drying to the skin, especially if used in an alcohol-based formulation.

Salicylic Acid

What: A beta-hydroxy acid (or BHA) derived from willow tree bark; used for its exfoliating (or peeling) qualities. Designed to loosen and soften plugged pores.

Pros: Especially good for the treatment of blackheads.

Cons: Limited usefulness unless paired with other active ingredients.

Benzoyl Peroxide

What: Perhaps the most commonly used active ingredient in OTC acne medications, benzoyl peroxide's unique attribute is that it penetrates the pore to kill bacteria within the oil duct. Comes in 2.5%, 5%, 7% and 10% concentrations, though lower strengths seem about as effective as higher ones, and tend to be less drying.

Pros: Consistently effective against almost all types of acne except the most severe and resistant strains. Widely available in creams, lotions, gels, masks, and cleansers, so it's relatively easy to find a brand and a formulation you like.

Cons: Can be excessively drying in certain formulations (particularly gels). Can also cause redness and flaking of the skin.

OTC Remedies for Butt Bumps

As we've seen, acne doesn't just attack the face. It can also develop on the buttocks, among other places. Most butt bumps erupt when your pores get clogged with perspiration, bacteria and dead skin cells—the perfect breeding ground for papule-inducing germs. If left untreated, those germs will continue to accumulate and soon transform your minimally inflamed papules into festering pustules.

The best solution? Acne treatments containing benzoyl peroxide, such as Clean and Clear Persa Gel and Oxy-10 Vanishing Acne Medication. These products not only help heal both papules and pustules by combating bacteria, but also have a drying effect, which can be beneficial if the skin on your buttocks is oily. If you have dry skin that is prone to flaking, however, opt instead for products containing salicylic acid such as Exact Pore Treatment Gel and Neutrogena Clear Pore Treatment. These should gently exfoliate your skin without causing undue dryness. To prevent future outbreaks, we often recommend the use of alpha-hydroxy or acne masks to keep the pores clear and unplugged. Finally, since the skin on your buttocks is thicker than the skin on your face, you can usually try products there that contain relatively high concentrations of active ingredients.

Prescription-Strength Medications

Due to recent advances in the field and the publicity surrounding "breakthrough" acne treatments, some relatively new prescription medicines are nearly as well known to the general public as OTC products that have been around for decades. Most people, however, don't possess the foggiest notion as to how and why these drugs produce such dramatic results. Nor do they typically understand that the effectiveness of certain medications often comes at a steep price, both in real dollars and in potential side effects. Our rule of thumb: Start mild before you go wild. By that, we mean that you—and your dermatologist—ought to begin treatment with the gentlest medicine capable of addressing your acne problems, and progress to stronger medications only if your condition fails to improve within a reasonable amount of time.

Prescription-strength medications, by the way, take longer to work than most patients think. Depending on the drug, visible improvement may not be forthcoming for several weeks—or for several months. Along the way, dosage may need to be adjusted, and drugs may need to be added to or deleted from your regimen, based on how your skin and your system react. All of which leads to the inescapable fact that one of the most crucial ingredients in any successful treatment program is: YOU. So stay patient, be flexible, and most important, be faithful in following your dermatologist's instructions regarding how and when to take the prescribed medications we are about to describe.

Topical Antibiotics

What: Lotions, creams, roll-ons, and pads prescribed chiefly for treatment of mild to moderate acne. Clindamycin and erythromycin are prescribed most often; tetracycline less often.

Pros: Topicals allow restriction of treatment to the problem area, so you don't have to expose your entire system to the drug, as with oral antibiotics. Also, they usually produce visible results in three to four weeks time, which is fairly quick for a prescribed medication.

Cons: Can cause excessive dryness of the skin, as well as burning, itching, stinging, inflammation, or flaking of treated region.

Oral Antibiotics

What: Drugs designed to treat moderate to severe acne by reducing inflammation of acne lesions. Often paired with topical antibiotics at the start of treatment, then gradually eliminated as topicals begin to produce positive results. Erythromycin, minocycline, tetracycline, and tetracycline derivatives are the most commonly prescribed oral antibiotics. Clindamycin is also occasionally prescribed, but only for very severe or persistent acne.

Pros: A time-tested way to successfully combat forms of acne that do not respond to topical treatment alone.

Cons: Visible results take anywhere from three to six weeks to appear. Possible side effects—which vary depending on the specific drug you take—range from stomach upset, queasiness, and diarrhea, to photosensitive reactions, headaches, and vaginal yeast infections. Also, many oral antibiotics must be taken on an empty stomach.

Retin-A™, Avita™

What: A mild, synthetic form of vitamin A acid (technically known as tretinoin) that serves as the active ingredient in various topical acne medications. These topical creams work by penetrating plugged pores to loosen thick, gummy cells, enabling them to be shed and thereby speeding up the cellular replacement cycle. Typically found in creams, lotions, and gels.

Pros: Not only clears up existing acne bumps, when effective, but also helps prevent the formation of new ones. In addition, some researchers believe that tretinoin renders the skin smoother, clearer, and less susceptible to wrinkling.

Cons: Can be drying and/or irritating to the skin, especially in gel formulations or when used in conjunction with other acne medications. May actually worsen your acne at first, or if the prescribed formulation is too strong. Makes your skin *more* sensitive to the sun.

Differin™

What: A topical retinoid product whose active ingredient (adapalene) dries and peels the skin to unclog plugged pores. Prescribed as a gel or solution.

Pros: Exfoliates as reliably as tretinoin, but without causing the redness that often results from using the more well-known medication. Especially effective for the treatment of pimples that erupt on the back. No increase in sun sensitivity.

Cons: Dryness and itching usually occur during the first two weeks of use. Must be used in combination with antibiotics for inflamed acne.

Ortho Tri-Cyclen™

What: An oral medication that acts as both a birth control pill and acne-fighting drug. Active ingredients are norgestimate and ethinyl estradiol, both of which are hormone-like substances used for their contraceptive qualities.

Pros: Regulates androgen production, making it ideal for breakouts linked to hormonal fluctuations. Doubles as birth control.

Cons: Prevents conception in those who want to take it solely for prevention of acne. Produces the side effects commonly associated with other oral contraceptives, such as skin discoloration, fluid retention, and spotting.

Accutane™

What: An extremely powerful oral medication prescribed for only the most severe, scarring types of acne. Like Retin-A™, its active ingredient (isotretinoin) is a vitamin A derivative.

Pros: Perhaps the closest thing we have to a true acne "cure." Extraordinarily effective in reducing sebum production by the oil glands and halting—sometimes permanently—the development of acne in those who use it.

Cons: MANY. We put this in caps because the side effects of Accutane™ for some patients can make even a very nasty case of acne seem like a small problem indeed. The complete list includes: excessively dry skin; dry, scratchy eyes; dry nose lining; dry mouth; sore muscles; stiff joints; headaches; impaired night vision; heightened cholesterol levels; increased production of liver enzymes; and severe birth defects in babies born to mothers who take the drug either shortly before conception or during pregnancy. Of course, not everyone—or even most people—will suffer the worst of these potential side effects. But you must be aware that they exist before you consider taking what amounts to a drug of last resort. One final note on Accutane™: Despite its strength, most prescriptions typically run a long time—4 to 5 months, on average.

Effective Medicines for Stubborn Bacterial Strains

Recently doctors made a jolting discovery: Certain strains of acne-causing bacteria have become resistant to many common antibiotics. These strains tend to creep up in people who frequently use antibiotics to treat their acne. The problem generally arises when the acne sufferer has either taken low dosages over a period of several years or has repeatedly initiated treatment in the past, only to give up before seeing results. In such cases, increasing the dosage of the current medication or switching to a new one will often help. The following drugs have proved especially effective in bringing resistant strains under control and, as a bonus, are usually less drying than conventional treatments. If the program you're on now doesn't appear to be working or has become ineffective over time, you might want to ask your dermatologist if one of them is appropriate for you.

Benzamycin™

What: An older topical drug that has recently been enjoying renewed popularity; active ingredients are benzoyl peroxide and erythromycin. Prescribed in gel or solution formulations.

Pros: Particularly effective in fighting those acne strains that have become resistant to other antibiotics, whether OTC or prescribed.

Cons: Though less drying than many comparable medications, benzamycin can cause dryness and skin irritation in some patients, especially if applied too generously.

Azalex™

What: A topical antibiotic cream that employs a derivative of wheat called azelaic acid to kill bacteria and reduce inflammation.
Pros: Good success rate in soothing and subduing inflamed lesions; sometimes even fades the brown or pink spots that often result at the sites of healed acne bumps. Less drying than comparable medications. Excellent for treating resistant strains.
Cons: Some patients experience hypopigmentation, or lightening of the skin, on treated areas.

Klaron™

What: A topical antibiotic cream with sodium sulfacetamide as the active ingredient.
Pros: Works effectively on resistant strains; comes in a water base that dries clear and is suitable for sensitive skin types.
Cons: Can cause adverse reactions such as stinging and burning in those allergic to sulfa drugs.

Triaz™

What: A topical peeling agent that features benzoyl peroxide in a glycolic acid and zinc base. Comes in gel form.
Pros: Benzoyl peroxide and glycolic acid in combination form a more effective pore declogger than either ingredient does on its own; can produce visible results within just two weeks. Also, zinc and other skin-soothing ingredients serve to minimize irritation. *Cons:* Must be used in conjunction with oral antibiotics to treat more severe acne cases.

Below:
Many over-the-counter products are helpful in treating acne.

PUMPING UP & BREAKING OUT

When body builders and other athletes ingest illegal steroids to reduce workout fatigue and build muscle mass, they're pumping up more than just their biceps. Heavy cases of acne usually result, too, due to the overabundance of androgens in the athlete's system. Of course, mere zits, no matter how severe, are the least of the steroid abuser's worries. Prolonged use of dangerous, black market substances such as human growth hormone and animal testosterone without strict medical supervision may cause irreversible liver damage that can ultimately lead to liver failure—and death. If you know people at your gym or have friends at school who take such substances, you should warn them that they are playing with fire. Though they probably already know this, a word from you just might bring them back to their senses.

MYTHS & MISCONCEPTIONS ABOUT ACNE

The instant you break out with a few zits, you will almost certainly receive loads of well-intentioned, but often misguided, advice as to what caused them and how to treat them. Acne, like the common cold, is one of those disorders that lends itself to intense speculation and discussion by the non-medical public. The reasons for this are understandable enough. First of all, nearly everyone suffers from acne sooner or later, just as nearly everyone comes down with a cold at some point. People feel as though they have experience with the problem, and therefore develop opinions about its causes and treatment. Second, since no definitive acne cure exists, all kinds of "home remedies" and therapies have been concocted over the years. Here again, the same holds true for the common cold, which people try to treat with everything from chicken soup to hot baths and heating pads. Finally, there is all too human temptation to assume that a person with acne has somehow "brought on" the disease by virtue of a poor diet, bad hygiene or sexual promiscuity, much in the manner that cold sufferers are assumed by some to have caught their colds by not dressing warmly enough in the winter. Of course, nothing of the sort is true in either case. We've already examined the main reasons and remedies for acne, and no reputable doctor would suggest that you catch a cold by getting cold (the real culprit is usually a viral or bacterial invader). Yet the myths and misconceptions persist.

Now, some of the myths surrounding acne are essentially harmless, but others most definitely aren't. In fact, we can pretty much guarantee that you'll worsen your acne if you follow certain bits of advice that have been floating around for ages. To help you avoid mistreatment, and to clear up any confusion you may have about the disorder, let's take a closer look at the most widespread of these popular myths.

Myth #1: Eating the wrong foods causes acne.
People who believe this myth will caution you to stay away from chocolate, fried foods and junk food snacks. Soda is also mentioned sometimes, but not as often as the others. Your diet, however, doesn't significantly increase or reduce your chances of developing acne, no matter how healthy or unhealthy it may be. Sure, you may experience a zit-like eruption due to a food allergy, but the cause for that type of breakout isn't restricted to junk foods. Any food could cause it, and junk foods aren't even among the worst offenders in sparking allergic reactions. But before you race to the nearest fast-food chain to order a triple cheeseburger, super-sized fries, and a milkshake, please bear in mind what these foods can do to your waistline and your arteries!

Myth #2: Dirt causes acne.
This is a deceptively dangerous myth because most of our readers, particularly here in America, are more likely to aggravate their acne through over-cleaning than by not cleaning frequently or thoroughly enough. As we've demonstrated, most cases of acne begin in the oil glands, which are *below the surface of the skin*. Superficial dirt and grime, then, simply aren't at the root of the problem, unless you happen to be very inattentive to personal hygiene.

Myth #3: Sex (or the lack of it) causes acne.
Contrary to what some mean-spirited people may suggest, acne is not the equivalent of a tabloid headline shouting: ZITS TELL

ALL! In fact, no direct connection exists between sexual activity and acne outbreaks.

Myth #4: The sun is good for acne because it dries up oily skin and creates a tan that helps hide unsightly blemishes.
This myth looks great on the surface, but is really rotten at the core. In fact, it wasn't so long ago that some dermatologists were recommending limited UV exposure as a means of clearing up acne. Shame on them—they should have known better! Although the sun can dry up and obscure pimples to an extent, the short-term aesthetic benefits are grossly outweighed by the long-term consequences of photoaging. What's more, UV rays have the effect of thickening epidermal cells, which can close off pores and actually worsen your acne problems.

Myth #5: Acne is a disease that afflicts teenagers only.
While it's true that acne affects teens more than any other age group, some forms of the disease are unique to adults, and some people suffer from chronic acne throughout their lifetime. The good news is that most of us will "outgrow" our zits as we enter adulthood; the bad news is that some of us will not.

ACNE & BLACK SKIN

Blacks, as a rule, are less prone to acne than lighter skinned people. However, they seem more susceptible to scarring and long-term darkening of the skin when they do break out. Because of this, black women should exercise extra caution in dealing with even minor flare-ups. See your dermatologist at the first sign of a breakout, and if you have large pores or oily skin, stay clear of the thick moisturizers and oil-based cosmetics that can clog pores. Instead, look for gently drying cleansers, and choose water-based cos-

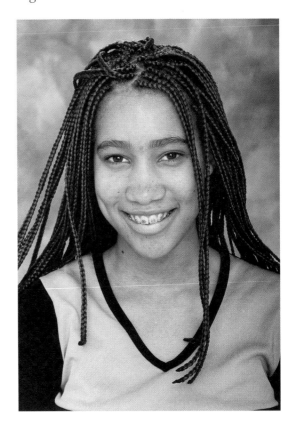

Below:
Black women have the advantage of fewer cases of acne, but even a slight breakout may lead to serious scarring and long-term darkening of the skin.

metics and skin care products that are both non-comedogenic and non-acnegenic.

ROAD RULES

Please Don't . . .

- *Pinch, rub, squeeze, or worst of all, ever pop a zit.* Now, we know there's something about a zit that simply cries out for popping. But no matter how small the blemish or how tempted you become: KEEP YOUR HANDS OFF! When you pop—or even merely rub—a zit, you nearly always increase the swelling, damage the surrounding skin, and heighten the risk of further bacterial infection. Most often, in fact, a popped whitehead or cyst will rupture beneath the pore, making it even more embedded and difficult to treat than it was before you took matters into your own hands. Unless you're very fortunate, permanent scarring is likely to result.

Below:

Always use a light touch when cleansing . . . vigorous scrubbing can lead to skin damage.

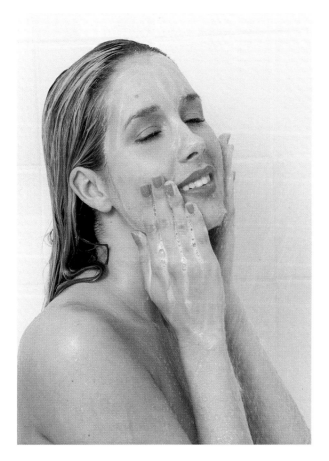

- *Overclean your skin.* Washing too often, too vigorously, or with overly harsh cleansers are mistakes that many acne sufferers commonly commit. The impulse is understandable enough. But since most acne cases stem from hormonal or hereditary causes, the results are usually ineffective at best and damaging at worst. Always remember that your distressed skin needs to be babied, not manhandled, especially if your acne is deeply embedded or cystic.

Please Do . . .

- Gently cleanse your skin at least twice daily with soap and water, using the guidelines we set forth in Chapter Two.
- Use water-based cosmetics, cleansers, and skin care products,

as opposed to oil-based products if your skin tends to be oily. If you're unsure after reading the label whether a certain item in your cosmetic bag is oil-based, put a dab on your fingertip, run some tap water on it, and try to rub it off. If the water beads up and the stuff stays put, you're probably dealing with an oil-based product. Products labeled as *non-comedogenic* or *non-acnegenic* are also usually wise choices for anyone with breakout-prone skin. This means that the item has been lab tested and does not produce pimples (non-comedogenic) or cause the formation of acne (non-acnegenic) when applied to normal skin.

- Drink plenty of water, which does a wonderful job of flushing impurities not only from the skin but from all of the body's organ systems as well.
- Eat a healthy diet that includes generous quantities of fresh fruits and vegetables. As you'll learn in Chapter Eight, foods that are rich in Vitamins A, C, and E are especially conducive to healthy, blemish-free skin.

END NOTES

1. Birth control pills achieve contraception by chemically simulating a false pregnancy within a woman's body. This deception is created chiefly by introducing androgen-like and estrogen-like substances of the type that normally flood an expectant mother's system soon after conception.
2. See, for example, makeup artist Bobbi Brown's excellent book, *Bobbi Brown Beauty*.

For more information on acne, go to
www.derm-infonet.com/acnenet/toc.html

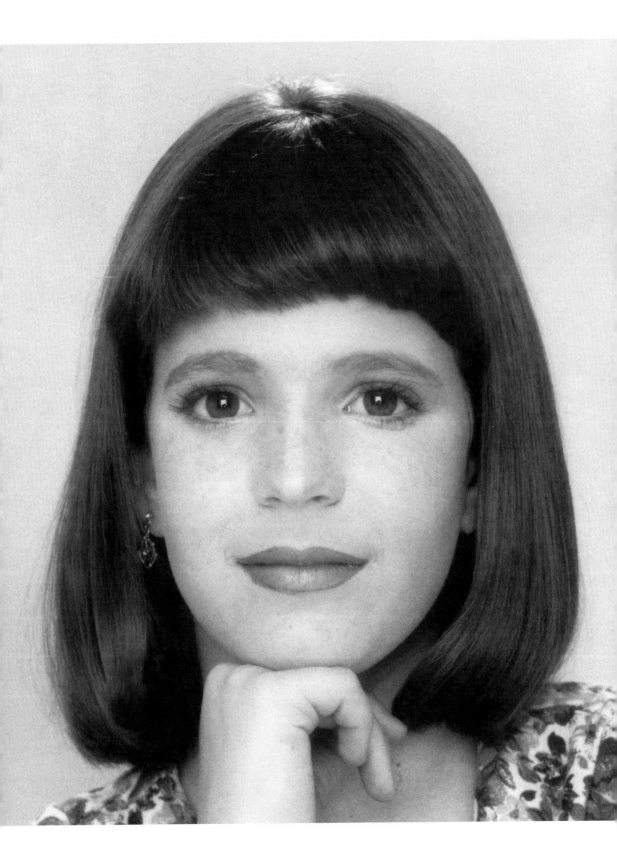

Going Straight to the Roots: Hair Structure, Hair Growth, & Hair Loss

Say the word "hair" and most of us instant-ly think of the stuff on top of our heads. Now, this is understandable enough. Human hair does tend to grow longer, thicker, and more plentifully on the scalp than elsewhere on the body. But the not-so-bald truth is that hair covers nearly every square inch of our face and body, no less thoroughly than if we were a chim-panzee or a gorilla. In fact, you'll find only a few truly hairless regions on the skin's surface. These areas include the palms of the hand, the soles of the feet, the fingertips, the eyeballs and the inside of the mouth. Look closely anyplace else and you'll see . . . hair, hair everywhere!

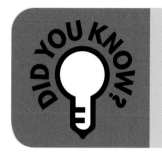

The top side of your tongue contains hair follicles that are perfectly capable of producing vellus hairs long enough to be seen by the naked eye. Blessedly, keeping those hairs under control and out of sight is no major deal: Just lightly brush your tongue with your toothbrush bristles every time you clean your teeth.

VELLUS HAIRS

The reason we *appear* less hairy than our close evolutionary relatives can be explained by hair types and how different types of hair are dispersed over the surface of the skin. In contrast to the body of a chimp, much of the human anatomy is covered by *vellus hairs*, which are remarkably short, fine, and colorless, rendering them in many locations all but invisible to the naked eye. Thus certain areas that seem to be hairless, such as the earlobes or the inside of the forearms, are actually coated by literally thousands of soft, downy vellus strands. In a word: hair!

Below:
Healthy hair can be one of your greatest beauty assets.

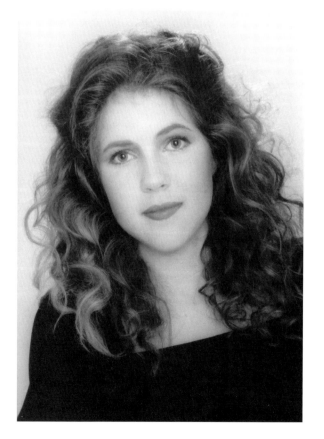

TERMINAL HAIRS

The hairs that you comb are examples of *terminal hairs*. Terminal hairs can be found on the scalp, face, armpits, eyelids (in the form of eyelashes), eyebrows, legs, and pubic regions. They are longer, thicker, and coarser than vellus hairs, and also contain melanin, which accounts for their coloring. Among terminal hairs, strands located on the scalp grow out more fully than strands covering, say, the extremities or the eyebrows, and even separate strands in the same general area will show variations in length, thickness, and curl. These variations are usually minor, but not always, which is why the hair strands on one portion of your head may "do the wave," while their neighbors lay quietly along the scalp.

A SINGLE STRAND OF HAIR

The visible portion of a hair strand, whether vellus or terminal, is not alive in the sense that the shampoo and conditioner ads would have you believe. Thus it cannot be "nourished," "rejuvenated," "invigorated," or made to thrive the way, for instance, a plant thrives in response to watering or fertilization. This is so because the living, reproductive portion of an individual hair strand resides deep below the skin's surface in a bulb-like sac called a follicle.[1] The part you see—and care for—is the hair shaft, which is composed of a non-living, fibrous protein known as *keratin*. Live cells within the hair root generate the shaft and sustain its subsequent growth.

The shaft itself is a two-piece affair, consisting of an outer, protective covering called the *cuticle*, and an inner, supportive nucleus called the *cortex*. In very basic terms, the cortex gives the hair strand its structure and strength, while the cuticle shields the cortex from the environment. When damage to the cuticle exposes the cortex to the elements, the affected hair becomes split or fractured. Too much washing, too much blow-drying, and overuse of the strong chemicals found in permanent wave solutions, straighteners, and other hair care products are just a few of the most common causes of dry, brittle hair that wants to fray and break.

HAIR GROWTH

Hair growth takes place in long cycles, each of which exhibits three distinct phases:
- a growing (or *anagen*) phase
- a resting (or *telogen*) phase
- a falling out (or *catagen*) phase

The growing phase lasts by far the longest of the three, occurring over two to five years in normal, healthy hair. Throughout this phase, fresh keratin is pumped from the bulb at the base of the follicle to the hair shaft, which not only promotes continued growth of the strand, but also reinforces it. Growth rates, of course, vary from one person to the next, but for most folks scalp

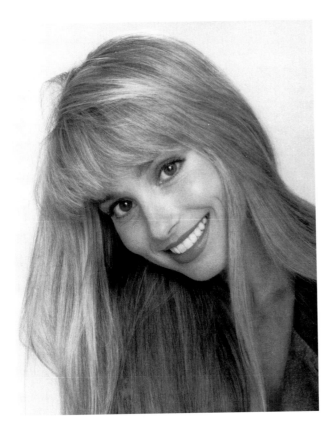

Above:
Healthy hair looks good at any length.

hair gains ½ to ¾ inch in length per month; body hair, around ¼ inch per month. The duration of the growing phase, incidentally, sets a physical limit on an individual's maximum hair length. A longer growth phase, as you'd expect, offers the potential for longer hair, though most of us have our hair cut too frequently to ever reach this biological threshold.

After the growing phase has ended, a brief resting phase of one to two weeks follows, then gives way, in turn, to a falling out phase of two to three months. On completion of the full cycle, the old hair strand is shed and replaced by a new one from the same follicle. Significantly, each strand has its own unique cycle, which is a good thing, if you think about it. Just consider: If all—or even most—of our follicles operated according to the same clock, we'd have to endure periodic bouts of heavy shedding and temporary baldness. Not a pleasant thought!

HAIR LOSS
Shedding: By the Numbers

At any one time, approximately 85% of the hair on your head is in the growing phase; the remainder, in the resting or falling out phases. While 85% may sound like—and in fact is—a lot, bear in mind that the remaining 15% represents a big number, too. The average person, you see, possesses somewhere between 60,000 and 130,000 scalp hairs. The exact number depends on the thickness of your hair and the concentration of follicles on your scalp: In general, people with fine hair tend to have more individual strands, people with coarse hair, relatively fewer. But either way, 15% of even 60,000 thick, coarse hairs means that

on any given day a minimum of 9,000 strands (or 60,000 ×
.15) are on the brink of cloggng your shower drain.

Of course, since the falling out phase is a two to three-month
process, you won't lose all 9,000-plus strands on the same day,
or even over the course of several weeks. *But you will shed at
least some hair every day*, and on some days noticeably more
than on others. So what's normal? 60 to 150 strands a day, on
average. The point here is that the hairs you see in the tub and
on your bathroom floor are there, more often than not, for good
reason: Your skin has ditched them to make room for healthy
new strands as part of the natural hair growth cycle.

But, Doctor . . . I See *Lots* of Hairs!

Despite these reassurances, we know from experience that some
teens will continue to freak over perfectly normal amounts of
hair loss. And while we hate to see them become unnecessarily
distressed, we'd much rather deal with people who are overly
concerned about the health of their skin and hair than with
those who don't care enough. So go ahead
and worry if you want, but don't just stew
over it: If you feel as though you're losing
more hair than you should, pick those
puppies up and count 'em. If the count
falls within the acceptable range of 150 or
less, you can rest easy. If it's higher, save
the hairs and bring them in to your dermatologist so that he or she can verify that
your count was correct[2] and, in the event
you are experiencing genuine hair loss,
test the strands to help determine the
cause of the problem.

The Most Common Causes
of Teen Hair Loss

We must preface our remarks about the
causes of teen hair loss by noting that true
hair loss—as opposed to normal shedding
or hair breakage—is exceedingly rare

Below:
*Even very thin hair can look
terrific with the right style.*

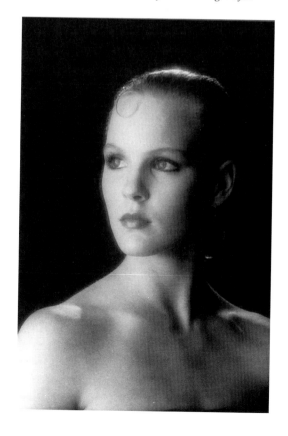

among teens of both sexes, and rarer still among teenage women. The reason you don't see high-school cheerleaders, female athletes, and 20-something women executives starring in the latest Hans Weiman and Rogaine™ commercials, after all, is that *men hold a near monopoly on baldness*. Further, when women do experience significant hair loss, it typically occurs after menopause and even then results in gradual thinning of hair, not the wholesale loss of coverage that afflicts so many men.[3]

The bottom line is that most of our readers are unlikely candidates for serious hair loss anytime soon. However, a small percentage of young women do suffer from hair loss disorders during their teen years. And while dozens of different conditions cause hair loss in the general population, just three strike this group with any degree of regularity. They are, in order of frequency of occurrence: trichotillomania, telogen effluvium, and alopecia areata. Let's take a look at all three conditions, one by one, and examine the symptoms associated with each.

Trichotillomania

Trichotillomania is a compulsive disorder in which the victim plucks and pulls out hairs to the point that significant hair loss ensues. You'll notice that we've used the word "victim" in describing people who suffer from this disease. On the surface, it might seem that someone who plucks out her own hair is somehow to blame for the problem, and that effecting a cure should be as simple as asking her to stop. But compulsive behavior differs in kind from normal behavior, so ordinary rules do not apply. People with this disorder are not dealing with an illness in the conventional sense of the term, but with something more on the order of a nervous tic.

Consequently, a person with trichotillomania can no more stop the hair-plucking behavior at the drop of a hat than someone with a repetitive facial tic can spontaneously stop it from twitching. The road to recovery therefore starts with acknowledging the problem and seeking treatment. Your dermatologist can address the hair loss associated with the condition, but curbing and controlling the compulsive behavior will probably require the services of a psychiatric or psychological specialist, since trichotillomania often stems from underlying emotional distress. Success rates for patients who receive treatment early on, by the way, are much higher than for those who postpone seeing their doctor and thus allow the behavior to become deeply ingrained. So if you believe you suffer from this disorder, please don't be afraid to seek help, and please don't wait. This is one problem that isn't likely to go away on its own.

Three Habits Worth Breaking: Chewing, Biting, & Playing With Hair

You may have observed that many children and teens engage in behaviors that slightly resemble trichotillomania, such as constantly chewing, biting, twisting, or twirling the hair. These types of nervous habits are very commonplace, especially among females, but are generally not compulsive in nature and thus do not usually require medical or psychiatric attention. They do, however, damage and distress the hair, causing split ends and fractured strands that do not stand up well to routine care, and cover poorly when brushed or combed. If you have a friend who habitually toys with her hair, we suggest that you politely bring it to her attention. In all likelihood, she isn't fully aware of what she's doing or how often she does it, and would be glad to know.

Telogen Effluvium

The second most common hair loss disorder among teenage women is *telogen effluvium*, which can be defined as stress-induced hair loss. The source of the stress can be either physical or psychological: On the physical side, typical triggers for the disorder include serious illness, a lengthy episode of high fever, starvation dieting, recent surgery, pregnancy, or termination of birth control. On the psychological side, the disease can be sparked by certain psychiatric conditions, the occurrence of a traumatic event, or eating disorders such as bulimia and anorexia nervosa. Telogen effluvium can take up to three months to develop fully, but when it does strike, the victim can hardly fail to notice it. In severe cases, up to 40 percent of the patient's hairs spontaneously shift from the growing phase to the resting phase,[4] prompting hair to fall out by the handful. In most cases, the condition subsides when the stress subsides, permitting the hair to regrow and revert to its normal growth cycle without extensive treatment. If the stress recurs, however, the disease can, too, so it's important to address any underlying causes that are within your control.

Alopecia Areata

Like the conditions we've just discussed, alopecia areata is rare among teens, but affects them more often than most other hair loss disorders. Its exact cause is unknown, but research suggests that it is an autoimmune disorder in which the body's natural defenses attack the hair roots as if they were a foreign substance or bacterial invader. The outcome: massive hair loss of the kind we saw with telogen effluvium[5]—and in extreme instances, total hair loss, including the loss of eyebrows, eyelashes, and pubic hair. More common, however, are comparatively milder cases, resulting in the appearance of round or oval hairless patches, which tend to spring up in pairs or in groups on different regions of the skin. Treatment, when given, generally centers around anti-inflammatory drugs such as corticosteroid creams, cortisone injections, and/or oral steroids, though the condition occasionally clears up on its own within a time frame of six to twelve months.

HAIR REMOVAL

Hair removal is an ongoing challenge faced by women of all ages—one that is at best annoying and time-consuming, and at worst, absolutely maddening and positively painful. But unless you let your bodily hair grow out or opt to have it permanently removed, there is no easy solution, despite what the makers of the latest hair removal product may claim in their ads. Hair, as we've seen, is supposed to grow all over your body. If it doesn't, you have a problem. You should therefore be skeptical of salons that promise "root destroying" waxing therapies or epilators that buzz hair away for keeps. They just don't work, at least beyond the short term.

Since there is no "magic bullet" for removing unwanted hair, your goal should be to make the process as quick, painless, and aesthetically pleasing as possible. Fortunately, many traditional and newer hair removal methods will allow you to do just that. The key is finding the right one for you, then deriving the best results from your chosen method. Here are some guidelines to help you get there.

Bleaching

If you're a stickler for precision, bleaching doesn't count as a true hair *removal* method. After all, the hairs are still in place when you're finished! But results are results, and a bleached hair that can't be seen is as good as gone from an aesthetic point of view. Bleaching, in fact, is a service offered at many fine salons, though it can easily be done at home, too, using any one of the commercial bleaches found in most drugstores and beauty supply stores.

The chief benefits of bleaching, assuming you do it yourself, are that it is inexpensive and doesn't leave you with stubble, as shaving sometimes does. Its usefulness, however, is limited to light-complected people. If you have brown, black, or even very tanned white skin, the contrast between your dark coloring and the bleached hairs will tend to make the hairs you're trying to hide more visible, not less. Bleaching is also something of a tricky art, in which timing is of the essence. Take the bleach off too soon and you wind up with red hairs; leave it on too long and you wind up with dry, irritated skin.

In case you can't tell, we're not the world's biggest fans of bleaching. But if you decide to try it anyhow, be sure to keep the product away from your eyes, mouth, and nasal passages. The lips, mouth, and nose are especially vulnerable when bleach is applied to the upper lip.

Below:
The eyes have it with well-groomed brows.

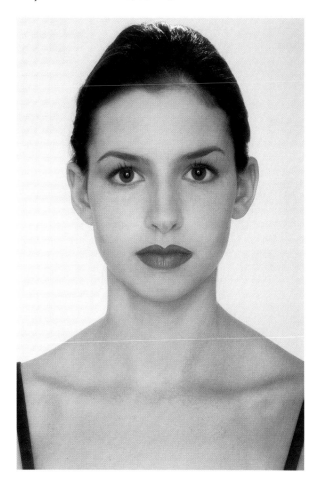

Plucking

Plucking, the preferred method for shaping the eyebrows, is exactly what it sounds like—removing hairs one by one with tweezers. You may have heard somewhere that plucked hairs do not grow back or that they grow back longer, darker, and coarser. Well, both notions are completely misguided. Your plucked hairs will regrow just fine. But you should still exercise caution when tweezing, since the growth cycle of eyebrow hairs (and eyelashes) is much, much shorter than that of your scalp hairs. Pluck too much at one sitting, and you may wind up with a thin, sparse look that won't appear full again for several weeks.

Some tips for plucking like a pro:

- Pluck selectively and slowly. Shaping your eyebrows gradually over the course of several days almost always delivers better results than doing the whole job at once.
- Use good-quality tweezers, and sterilize them frequently. Papules, pustules, and ingrown hairs can develop in the pores of plucked sites, so you want to keep your equipment clean to minimize the risk of infection.
- Angled tweezers work best for most people most of the time. Pointed tweezers, on the other hand, require more skill to use, and have a tendency to snap the shafts of longer hairs. Two brands we've used and liked: Revlon and Tweezerman, the latter available in hot pink (what a hoot!).

Shaving

As with plucking, shaving will not cause your hair to grow back thicker, darker, or longer. A clean, close shave typically lasts one to three days, depending on how quickly your hair grows and how manic you are about stubble. Your biggest decision here is pretty obvious: hand-held safety razor or electric? We don't recommend one over the other, but convention-

Below:

Shaving is the most popular method of hair removal for sensitive areas.

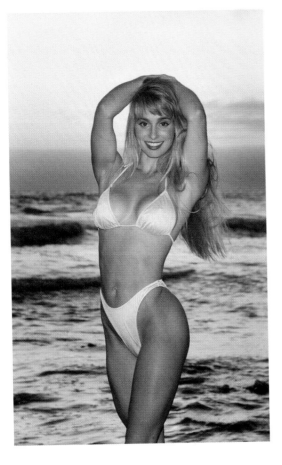

al wisdom says to use a safety razor if closeness is your priority, an electric if comfort is your aim. Some tips for using both:

For Safety or Electric Razors

- Don't try to shave immediately after bathing; your skin will be puckered and the results will be uneven.
- For a cleaner look, always cut against the grain of the hair growth. You'll break the hair shafts closer to the skin's surface that way.
- After you shave, rinse all shaved areas thoroughly with water, but wait a while before applying soap, deodorant or antiperspirant, all of which can make freshly shaved skin burn and sting.
- To prevent ingrown hairs on shaved skin, exfoliate gently with lotions and creams containing alpha-hydroxy acids between shaves.

For Safety Razors

- Isn't it ironic that a so-called "safety" razor is the one that tends to nick and cut? To reduce the potential for damage, always start with a clean, sharp razor. Odd as it may sound, a sharper blade is less likely to nick you, because it cuts cleanly. Dull blades tend to snag and gouge. Ouch!
- Hydrated hair is easier to cut, so rinse in warm (not scalding) water two to three minutes prior to shaving, then apply shaving cream—or in a pinch, hair conditioner—to retain the moisture. If razor bumps are a problem for you, let the shaving cream stand for a couple of extra minutes before shaving.

For Electric Razors

- Wet skin will make your electric razor want to stick and grab, resulting in a poor, uneven cut, so start off right by making sure your skin is completely dry before shaving.

Chemical Depilatories

Depilatories are creams, lotions, and gels that sever hair just below the skin's surface by chemically dissolving the strong sulfur bonds that try to keep your hair shafts in one piece. Lotions and gels are designed for use on the body; creams, for use on the face. Gentler on the skin than shaving or waxing, depilatories are especially good for sensitive or bumpy areas such as the bikini line, the upper lip, and the underarms. Plus, the results last for a week or more, so you'll save yourself some time in the maintenance department, versus shaving.

In theory, a depilatory should render your skin smoother than shaving, because the chemical process breaks hair off below the skin's surface. In practice, we find that women offer mixed opinions: Some prefer the look of razor-shaved skin; others swear by their cream or gel. Also, some depilatories can prove irritating to the skin, especially if you have sensitive skin or use the wrong formulation in the wrong place. To play it safe, alway apply a smattering of an untried product on a small test area to see how your skin reacts. If redness or stinging occur, you may need to switch to a different hair removal method, select a different brand of depilatory, or change to a gentler formulation. On the whole, creams will be gentler than lotions, lotions gentler than gels.

Some to try: Sally Hansen's Sponge-On Hair Remover, Nair 3-In-1 Lotion, Nair Cream Hair Remover For Face, and Nair Roll-On (great for legs!).

Waxing

Waxing removes hair at or near the root, and so will keep your skin hairless for four to eight weeks at a time[6] when done properly. In this process, a thin layer of warm or cold wax is applied to the skin and then stripped off, thus tearing unwanted hairs out of their follicles. Warm waxes are applied in a melted, semi-liquid state; cold waxes (which are generally sold as adhesive strips), straight from the package.

The main advantages of waxing are twofold: first, you spend far less time on maintenance than with any other conventional hair removal method; and second, the resulting look is exceptionally clean and smooth. On the down

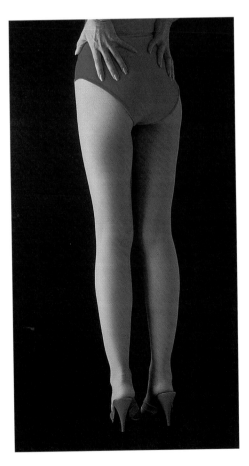

Below:
Waxing produces a long-lasting, smooth finish for your legs and bikini area.

side, waxing can not only be somewhat painful, but can also prove difficult to do well at home because a certain degree of dexterity is required. In addition, you must allow the hairs to grow out at least ¼ inch above the skin surface before waxing again, a length some women find unacceptable, even for short periods of time.

For those who swear by waxing, the critical question is whether to do it at home or go to a salon. The salon route, of course, is the more expensive of the two: Rates will vary from place to place, but typical salon pricing runs from about $10 for an eyebrow treatment, to $50 and up for legs. Most aestheticians, by the way, like to use hot wax, so you'll probably need to request cold wax if you have sensitive skin or simply prefer cold wax to hot.

If salons are too pricey or just not your style, several at-home kits will allow you to remove plenty of hair for under $10. The best of the best:

- Marzena Genuine Wax Strips. No mess, no fuss, just press and pull. The Petite Strips are great for your bikini line and facial hair; the Leg Strips, for areas where more coverage is needed. Available at many beauty supply, drug, and grocery stores, or by calling 1-800-380-3386.
- My-epil's Cold Wax Strips or Sally Hansen's Hair Remover Wax Strip Kit. Both come packaged against a sheet of cellophane, so you don't have to touch the sticky stuff at all. Nice goods; and cheap to boot, at under $10 each.[7]
- Nair Salon-Style Wax Kits. Easy to find and easy to use; available in both warm and cold varieties.

Some Like It Hot . . .

Hot wax usually comes in a tub, and remains hard until heated. For best results, heat the product according to the manufacturer's instructions; then apply a thin, even coat where desired, using a wooden tongue depressor. Remove wax as it cools, with a clean cotton washcloth to lift hairs. Since you can't allow the wax to get cold on your skin, work on one limited area at a time, and be sure you have everything you need at hand. Finally, remember that your first efforts will probably not be your best, because applying the wax skillfully takes a little practice (that's why women go to salons). But stick with it: Your third or fourth try will generally give you a much better idea than the first of the results you can expect going forward.

And Some Like It Cold

Though hot waxes are considered the big challenge for at-home use, cold wax kits require nimble fingers, too. When working with them, keep these simple guidelines in mind: (1) follow the instructions on the package to the letter; (2) do your level best not to handle the tacky side of the strip; (3) peel the strip back from the top—don't pull up—when you remove it; and (4) screw up your courage and peel the strip back quickly—like when you remove a well-stuck Band-Aid, it's more efficient and less painful that way.

Permanent Hair Removal Methods

The permanent removal of hair is hard work for both the patient undergoing treatment and the technician who treats her. Currently, three methods of permanent hair removal are practiced: *electrolysis, thermolysis,* and *laser epilation.* Electrolysis involves zapping hair follicles with electricity; thermolysis, with heat; and laser epilation, with an intensely concentrated beam of light. All three methods seek to kill the live cluster of cells (called the *hair matrix*) responsible for the generation of hair roots.

Sounds easy, you say? Well, trust us, it's not! Hair, as you'll recall, grows in cycles, and only a follicle with a growing hair in it can be treated successfully. So the permanent removal of all hairs in an area, even a very small one, can require several treatments. Beyond that obstacle, each hair matrix within the treated area must be destroyed one by one. A trained technician must insert a tiny probe into the hair follicle with a high degree of precision, or the job—for that particular follicle at least—is botched. To get an idea of how much work this entails, pretend that you want the hair on your upper lip removed (a common request), then look in the mirror and start counting the follicles. You can stop at around 300, because that's how many a really good technician will be able to treat in a single session.[8]

All of this slow, painstaking work, of course, comes at a price. Treatment costs range from approximately $35 per visit for electrolysis, to several hundred dollars a pop for laser therapy. And since treatment usually takes place over a series of sessions, the final tab can easily reach into thousands of dollars. Treatment can also exact a physical toll on the patient, especially when it is performed on sensitive facial regions. Many women find the prickly, snapping sensations caused by these procedures to be painful, and some women experience slight scarring around the treated follicles. Many others, however, consider the discomfort to be minimal, and do not scar at all.

Electrolysis & Thermolysis

In both of these methods, a technician inserts a wire-like probe, called an epilating needle, into the hair follicle until it reaches the follicle base, where the matrix resides. Once the probe has been successfully inserted, electrical current (electrolysis) or heat (thermolysis) is transmitted through the needle to scorch the matrix. When performed correctly, both procedures are extremely effective at eliminating unwanted hairs—not just for now but forever. You will, however, need to be patient: Remember that even the best technician cannot zap hairs in the resting phase, and that it takes real time to cover all the follicles in a given area. For the most commonly requested procedures, figure on a minimum of six to eight monthly treatments before you start seeing the results you want, somewhat more if you're having extensive work done.

If you elect to pursue either of these hair removal methods, do yourself a huge favor and have the treatments done by the most gifted, experienced technician you can find. Good "techs" will save you time (they work fast and so get the job done in fewer visits), money (you're paying by the visit), and scars (they don't misplace the probe or scorch your skin with too much juice). Plus, you'll wind up with smooth, hair-free skin that may never feel the edge of a razor again. A bad tech, on the other hand, can be your worst beauty nightmare. At the very least, you want a board-certified technician who works with computerized, digital equipment, and uses disposable, insulated probes.[9] A better option, though, is to talk to your dermatologist and ask him to give you the name of the best technician within driving distance of your home. An established dermatologist will typically have a well-formed, professional opinion about whom you should see, and that's always a great starting point for your search.

Laser Epilation

This method is most recommended by the medical community, and the FDA (Food and Drug Administration) has approved almost a dozen laser hair removal systems for use in the U.S.[10] We should note, however, that *current laser systems cannot claim or guarantee permanent hair removal* just yet, although they've been in use for a few years. But the early signs are promising: Regrowth rates in patients treated with today's technology have tended to drop with each successive treatment, and new procedures offering the prospect of permanent removal appear to be just around the corner.

The most popular FDA-approved systems currently in use are the following:

- **The ruby laser** heats and ultimately destroys the hair root with intense laser light energy. The heat generated by this type of laser can be painful, so cooling tips are used on the probe to blunt the burning sensation. Another significant drawback of the ruby laser is that

Below:
Hair removal with a long-pulsed ruby laser.

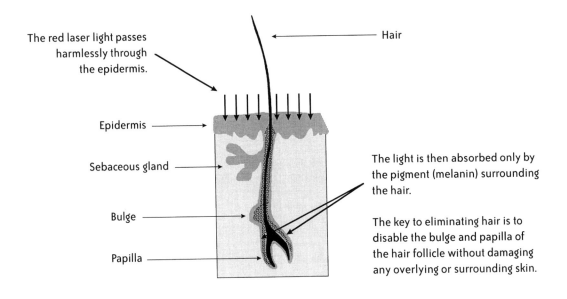

The red laser light passes harmlessly through the epidermis.

Hair

Epidermis

Sebaceous gland

Bulge

Papilla

The light is then absorbed only by the pigment (melanin) surrounding the hair.

The key to eliminating hair is to disable the bulge and papilla of the hair follicle without damaging any overlying or surrounding skin.

darker skinned persons have a tendency to develop white scars as a result of the procedure. Physicians, at least for the time being, must therefore restrict its use to light skinned patients only.

- **Alexandrite lasers** are often used to treat larger areas like the legs and back because they remove hair faster than the ruby laser. Although these systems have been

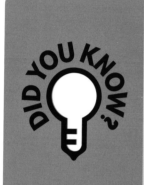

Lasers & Removal of Tattoos

Most of the laser systems used for hair removal can also be used, but at different settings, to eliminate unwanted tattoos, birthmarks, and other patches of dark pigmentation. The ruby laser, in fact, was not initially designed to remove hair. That step came only after doctors noticed that hair regrowth seemed to be delayed in regions where tattoos had been zapped by the concentrated beam of the laser. You should understand, however, that laser removal of a tattoo is neither cheap, quick, nor risk-free. A tattoo that cost you $100 to put on can easily cost upward of $2,000 to take off, and there is no guarantee that you won't wind up with scars, especially if the tattoo is multicolored or engraved deeply into the skin. Several separate treatments are necessary in most cases and depending on the colors used in the offending image and the equipment your doctors owns, more than one type of laser may need to be used.

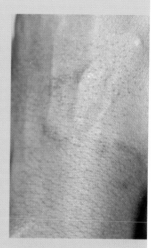

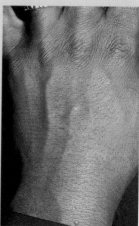

Above:

If your tattoo turns out not to be for you, no problem! Laser tattoo removal is the answer.

used with some success on dark skin, most dermatologists confine their usage to medium-complected patients.

- **The Epilight system** directs an intense light pulse to the hair root to heat and destroy it. This system is quick, relatively painless, and, like the alexandrite laser, good for regions that require broad coverage. However, it too works best on light- to medium-skinned patients. A newer Epilight system has shown the potential to work effectively on darker skinned people, but is still under evaluation.

- **The diode laser** was developed as a less painful alternative to early lasers. Like the ruby laser, the diode laser works relatively slowly, and has a cooling tip on the epilating needle to minimize patient discomfort. Among the currently approved systems, this one is the most effective for use on dark skin.

Before leaving the subject of permanent hair removal methods, we need to mention that these procedures should be avoided—or at the very least, approached with caution—by anyone who is susceptible to dark spots, or hyperpigmentation. Patients with this condition are often predisposed to suffer the scarring and localized skin discoloration that sometimes results from electrolysis, thermolysis, and laser therapy.

Below:

Why do blondes have more fun? They have more hair— it's a fact!

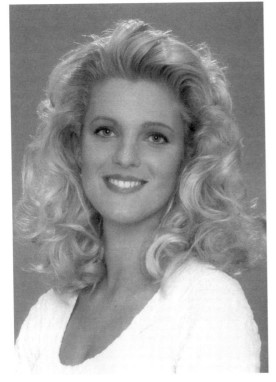

WHERE DID I GET THIS HAIR?

The short answer: from good old Mom and Dad. In fact, nearly all of the distinguishing features of your hair—its length, texture, thickness, shape, coloring, and curl—are inherited traits. Now that you know the scoop, we'll let you decide whether your parents should be thanked, or blamed, for the results!

Blondes Have More . . . Hair!

It's a fact: When it comes to the number of scalp hairs, blondes top the charts at 120,000 to 130,000 per head. Why? Because blonde hair tends to be thinner

Here's a statement you may have heard before: The only dumb question is the one you're afraid to ask. Corny, we admit. But true—especially as it pertains to excessive hair growth, or the appearance of dark body hairs in areas where you'd just as soon not see them. To spare you the discomfort of raising these questions yourself, we'll ask (and answer) them for you. Since our list isn't even close to being all-inclusive, don't be surprised if you have a question we haven't addressed. But don't keep yourself in the dark, either! We will happily answer any and all reader questions by e-mail. Our address is MGDERM@aol.com.

Q: *Help! I'm covered with so much dark hair, I look like a boy! What can I do?*

A: Hirsutism, or excessive hair growth, especially in women, is signaled by the appearance of dark, coarse hairs on the upper lip, chin, sideburns, chest, back, abdomen, and thighs. In basic terms, women with this condition grow terminal hairs in places where most women grow vellus hairs. The disease is hormonally based, and results from one or both of the following causes:

- overproduction of male sex hormones (androgens)
- hypersensitivity (= oversensitivity) of the hair follicles to normal androgen levels

As you can imagine, hirsutism represents both a medical and an emotional problem for most of the women afflicted by it—thanks mainly to our conventional notions of feminine beauty and the negative way in which society views women who display so-called male characteristics. Unfortunately, no FDA-approved medication presently exists to reverse or cure the disorder on a permanent basis. As a result, therapy focuses almost exclusively on the cosmetic issue of eliminating the unwanted hair. The starting point, for most patients, will be prescription medications designed to suppress androgen production, though many hirsute women nowadays also choose to supplement their drug therapy with electrolysis, laser or pulsed-light hair removal treatments.

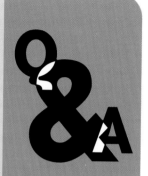

YOU HAVE HAIR *THERE*?

Answers to Questions You've Been Too Embarrassed to Ask

Q: *I have a few hairs around my nipples. Is this normal? And is it OK to pluck them?*

A: Yes on both counts, but be prepared to wince when you pluck—that's a tender spot!

Q: *I have a little red bump on my butt that looks and feels like a fresh mosquito bite. What is it? And how can I make it go away?*

A: Most likely, what you have is an ingrown hair. Everybody gets one every now and again, but those of us with wiry, kinky hair are generally most susceptible. An ingrown hair results when an individual hair grows back in a curve toward the skin, causing the free end to become lodged in a neighboring pore. The bumpiness, redness, and tenderness you've noticed tell us that the area around the hair has become slightly infected and inflamed, which is very common and probably no big deal.

To dislodge the ingrown hair, try scrubbing the affected area gently with a loofah sponge or synthetic pouf while you shower. If that fails, an over-the-counter alpha-hydroxy acid (AHA) cream (Estee Lauder Resilience Body, and Mary Kay Visible-Action Skin Revealing Lotion are two to try) or a prescribed cream containing Retin-A may open up that sore old pore. Last, if you'd like to prevent the problem from coming back to bite you, make either the loofah or the AHA cream part of your regular cleansing routine.

Q: *My new bikini is cut really small and I'm embarrassed by the dark line of hair running from my navel into the swimsuit bottom. Can this be fixed?*

A: Yes. In fact, we can offer three different fixes: one short, one medium, and one long-term. The short-term fix is to bleach the offending hairs; the medium-term fix, to wax them; the long-term fix, to eliminate them altogether with electrolysis or laser treatments. If it were us, though, we'd probably do bleach or wax, depending on the length and darkness of the hair in question. If the hair is light and fine, we'd bleach, provided we didn't have a really deep tan. If dark and long, we'd wax. As for the electrolysis or laser action, we'd only go there if we wore our swimsuit nearly every day throughout the year.

Q: *I can't stand to see hair anywhere around the line of my swimsuit. Can I handle this at home? Or do I need to visit a salon? Or my dermatologist's office?*

A: Basically, you can achieve your goal at any of these places. Stay home if you'd like to save some money. Head to the salon if you want the smooth, clean, and relatively long-lasting look of a professionally applied wax treatment. See your dermatologist if you want the area hair-free for life.

Of the three options, we'd advise that you try the at-home solution first, using the depilatory lotion or cream of your choice to do the job. Use of a depilatory strikes us as the right method for the broad—and in some places tender—area in question, for a number of reasons. First of all, a depilatory is quick and easy to apply, a major plus for removing hair from the hard-to-reach, hard-to-see spots you'll have to hit, like the lower back and inner thighs. Second, it provides a nice, clean look. And third, it keeps you hairless for a week or better—not as long as waxing, to be sure, but longer than bleaching or shaving. Other at-home methods, by contrast, seem to us too troublesome and too time-consuming to be practical for this specific purpose.

If you try a depilatory and it doesn't deliver the results you want, we'd suggest a visit to a salon or your dermatologist as a logical next step. Which of the two you choose will depend on how much you're willing to spend and the type of solution you're after.

than other shades. Your typical redhead, in comparison, has a paltry 60,000 to 90,000 strands, give or take, to call her own.

How Your Hair Gets (and Loses) Its Color

Your natural hair color is determined by melanocytes, or pigment-producing cells, that live at the base of every terminal hair follicle and supply pigment to one particular strand of hair. These cells function independently of each other, which helps explain why people usually turn gray gradually (the familiar "salt and pepper" look) rather than in a single fell swoop. Women, luckily for them, are far less susceptible to premature graying than men are. That means you probably have until your 30s, or possibly even your 40s or early 50s, before those pigment cells start thinking about retirement.

Summertime Blondes . . .

Many people who wish they were blonde see their dream come closer to reality over the course of the summer. Ever wonder why? Well, the reason is that UV exposure saps pigment from the hair shafts on your scalp, thus lightening their color. Now, if that were the end of the story, we could all go home happy. But those same UV rays also rob your hair shafts of their natural oils, which leaves the hair dry, brittle, and prone to break. Just one more reason to invest in a good, tightly woven (remember?) hat!

And You Thought Scary Movies Made Your Hair Curl!

The degree of waviness or curl in your hair is created by two kinds of chemical bonds: hydrogen bonds, which are relatively weak and can be broken down by mere wetting and combing; and sulfur bonds, which are stronger and require chemicals like those found in many hair care products to be broken. In addition, the shape of the hair shaft influences how straight or wavy a given hair will be. Most people assume that an individual hair shaft forms a nice round cylinder, and indeed that's the way you'll typically find one illustrated in a textbook. But in reality, the shape of the hair shaft varies by hair type. Straight hairs tend to have round shafts; wavy hairs usually have oval shafts; and curly or kinky hairs have a more flat, oval shaft. A wavy or curly hair, interestingly enough, begins to bend back and forth right at the base of the follicle—before we even have a chance to see it. The space separating each bend determines whether the resulting growth appears as a long, flowing wave, a close, springy curl, or something in between. As common sense suggests, a shorter space between bends produces more pronounced waves and tighter curls.

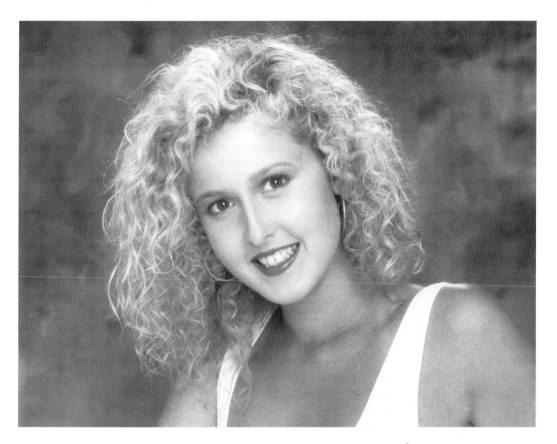

Above:

If you weren't born with curly locks and you want them, a trip to the drugstore or your favorite salon can produce results that would fool even your mom or your best friend!

END NOTES

1. Hair follicles originate at various depths. Some are located near the floor of the dermis, others near the top of the subcutaneous layer.

2. Concerned patients often mistake broken hairs for hairs that have been shed. After viewing the samples you bring in, your dermatologist should be able to tell you whether your hair is actually falling out or is merely brittle and prone to breakage.

3. Sadly, the very infrequency of the condition among teenage women is probably what makes many of them dread it so. No one likes to be singled out because of their appearance, and our culture simply does not yet accept female hair loss as openly and freely as it does male baldness.

4. Or telogen phase, hence the name of the disorder.

5. Another similarity between the two disorders is that stress is believed to sometimes play a role in the development of alopecia areata.

6. The roots of waxed hairs are usually destroyed, and it takes approximately a month for the follicle to generate a new root and start growing hair again.

7. All prices listed in this book reflect the current suggested retail at the time of writing. They do not include tax, and, of course, may vary somewhat from the prices you pay depending on when and where you shop.

8. The average regrowth rate for hair follicles treated with electrolysis or thermolysis is about 40 percent. Laser epilation is not yet advanced to the point of permanently removing hairs, but presently great strides are being made in that direction.

9. To find a qualified electrologist in your area or to confirm an operator's board certification, call the American Electrology Association at 203-374-6667.

10. To find a qualified, board-certified doctor for laser hair removal, you should contact the American Society for Dermatologic Surgery by calling 847-330-9830 or on the internet at www.asds-net.org, or the American Society of Laser Medicine and Surgery, 2404 Stewart Square, Wansan, WI 54401, 715-845-9283, Fax: 715-848-2493, Email: aslms@dwave.net.

For more information on hair loss, go to
http://cpmcnet.columbia.edu/dept/derm/hairloss/index.html

NOTES

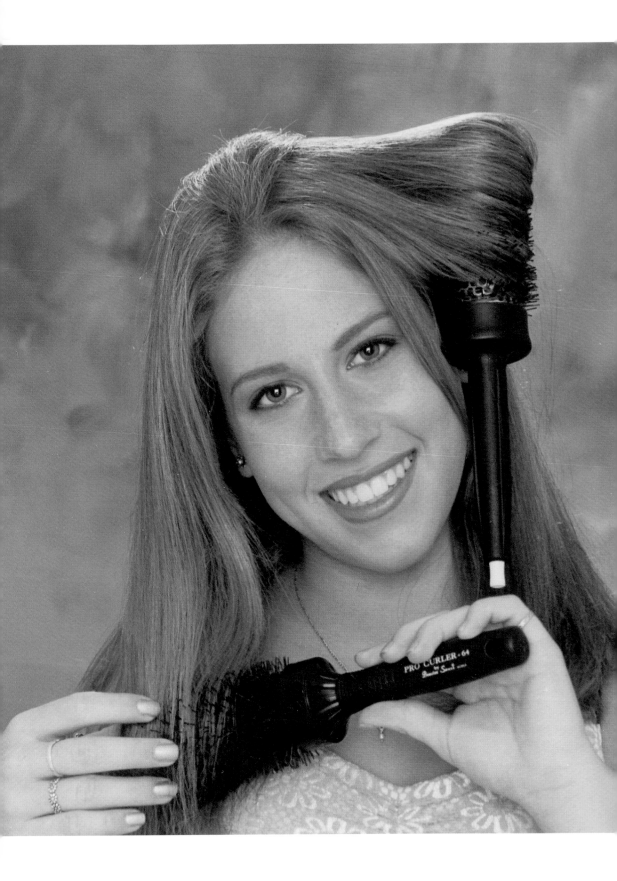

Have a Good Hair Day, *Every Day:* Hair Care, Hair Treatments, & Hair Styling

The cardinal rule of hair care and hair styling can be summed up in a single phrase: Work with what you've got. Sounds simple enough on paper, but putting it into everyday practice can be positively maddening. The biggest problem, of course, is that the hair we want generally bears zero resemblance to what's actually on top of our head. No, the hair we *really* want is most often found on the natural blonde who sits to our left in third-period algebra or—as rotten luck would have it—on the woman walking *into* the hairstyling salon just as we happen to be walking *out.*

In fairness, though, we can name at least three places where the hair we want can almost never, ever be found:

1. On our hairstylist's head (and this concerns us)
2. On our mother's head (can you say "genetics?")
3. On our own head (unless, of course, we were to be marooned on a remote desert island, in which case our hair would look flawless 24 hours a day, 7 days a week, just to spite us)

Jokes aside, the great majority of bad hair days occur because we've either rendered our hair unmanageable through improper use of hair care and styling products, or tried to impose a style on it that doesn't mesh with its natural tendencies. Happily, both mistakes can be avoided by adopting a sensible hair care regimen, then choosing a style that not only works within the limitations but also highlights the best features of our own humble head of hair. To accomplish these goals, we must first define the qualities that make hair appear healthy and beautiful.

Below:
There are four characteristics of fabulous hair: volume, lustre, length, and softness. This picture says it all.

CHARACTERISTICS OF GREAT LOOKING HAIR

Despite the changeable trends that make one color or one type of cut the popular favorite of the day, great-looking hair has always come in an endless variety of shades, styles, and textures.

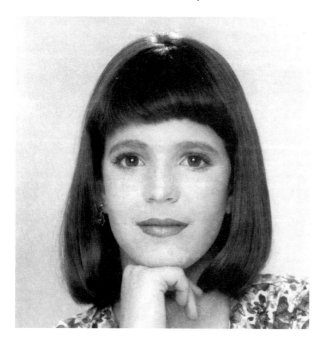

Sadly enough, the two characteristics of hair that women seem to obsess over the most—namely, color and curl—are also among the hardest to alter because they are inherited traits, as we learned in Chapter Five. Our own view is that you should see what magic you can work with your hair's natural color and texture before you resort to processes such as dyeing, waving, or straightening, all of which involve harsh chemical treatments that not only undermine hair health but also require constant upkeep (if you do it yourself) or expense (if your hairdresser or stylist does it for you). We will have more to say on the subject of chemical treatments later, but for now, let's examine those characteristics of hair that can be improved through intelligent, yet routine care. By our count, there are four such characteristics: volume, lustre, length, and softness. Get these right, and you'll be well on your way to a succession of good hair days.

Volume

The impression of hair volume—or fullness—is created by the thickness, not the total number, of individual hair strands you possess. The way this works in practice seems to defy common sense: Those of us with fewer hairs typically tend to enjoy a fuller look because the individual strands are thicker; and those of us with more hairs often have to cope with a sparser look because the individual strands are thinner.[1] So in this particular case, you could accurately say that "less is more," at least in terms of how full your hair appears.

Since we possess all the hair follicles we will ever own at birth, the only way to achieve a fuller look is to plump up individual strands artificially so that they appear thicker than they really are. And though the diameter of a hair shaft cannot be permanently enlarged, certain hair care products do cause it to swell temporarily. These include protein-rich shampoos, protein-rich conditioners, volumizers, and hair dyes, all of which not only bind chemically to the exterior of the shaft and thus fatten it, but also saturate the shaft internally for a short-term plumping effect.

Because body-building hair care products are generally effective at enhancing fullness, it's tempting to race straight to the drugstore to pick up something that you hope will "pump up the volume." A quick cure is always so appealing! However, a trade-off is involved: What you gain in fullness by using these products can often be more than offset by what you lose in terms of lustre, length, and softness, as we'll see momentarily. Here's why: Even the healthiest head of hair is composed of *nonliving* material, and so lacks the recuperative powers of the skin, which receives a constant flow of nutrients, water, and oxygen by way of the bloodstream. Your hair, then, is extraordinarily

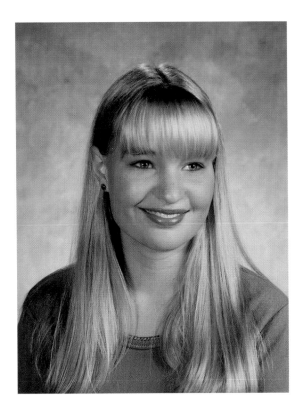

Above:
Shine on!

sensitive to—and easily damaged by—the chemicals that come in contact with it. As a result, you'll want to exercise both caution and moderation in choosing the number and types of products you use on a regular basis.

Lustre

Lustre, or shine, describes the glossy, vibrant appearance of healthy, undamaged hair. The key word in the previous sentence is "undamaged." In healthy hair, the cuticle covering that protects the cortex presents a smooth, even surface of interlocking, transparent cells.[2] Such a surface is ideal for reflecting light, and thus produces the attractive "lustre" or "radiance" that shampoo and conditioner manufacturers would like you to believe occurs solely from using their products. Natural oils on the hair shaft also promote lustre by filling in miniscule cracks, chips, and other irregularities on the surface of the cuticle. The cells of stressed or damaged hair shafts, on the other hand, form a jagged, uneven surface. This type of surface tends to swallow up light rather than reflect it, resulting in hair that lacks lustre and thus appears dull and lifeless. The built-up residue from sprays, setting lotions, mousses, gels, dyes, and other hair care products can also diminish shine by attracting tiny flecks of dust, dirt, grit, and grime, which attach themselves to the cuticle and thereby exaggerate existing surface irregularities.

While conditioners, low pH shampoos, and pH-balanced shampoos can all help to restore your hair's lustre by filling in the cracks and crevices of damaged hair shafts, it's important to note that the improvement is temporary and strictly cosmetic. Here again, keep in mind that hair does not function like live tissue. Once a shaft has become damaged, it's damaged for keeps—or at least until it has been shed and replaced by a plump, healthy new hair from the same follicle.

Length

An individual's hair length, as we observed in the previous chapter, has a biological limit imposed on it by the duration of the hair growing (or anagen) phase, which is determined by genetic inheritance and therefore cannot be changed. Many external factors, however, can snip inches off your hair's natural growth potential. Dry, brittle hairs typically fray or break long before they are shed, frequently as a direct consequence of excessive shampooing, overly aggressive blow-drying, or misuse of common hair care and hairstyling products.

To maximize hair length, you need to rein in the understandable—but all too often disastrous—desire to "make" your hair look gorgeous. That means giving the hair a day off from all hair care products from time to time, just as you should give your nails an occasional respite from polish. Some other sound practices, which we will later discuss in more detail, include gentle brushing and combing, sensible washing, low heat blow-drying, regular scalp massage, and sparing use of chemical treatments of all kinds.

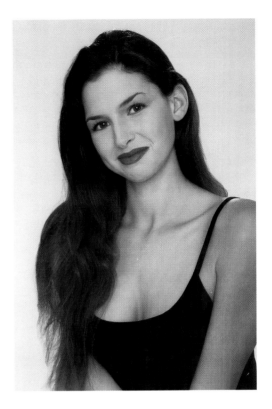

Above:
Blow-drying and styling products take their toll; for healthy hair at any length, give it an occasional rest from your daily routine.

Softness

Softness and flexibility are characteristics of hair that knows how to hang on to the moisture that keeps the keratin cells in your hair shafts fat and sassy. A plump, water-laden keratin cell is a happy keratin cell, and it rewards its owner with hair that is bouncy, soft to the touch, and easy to manage. When your hair is soft and flexible, even a strand that has been shed will still stretch, rather than snap, if you grasp both ends and pull in opposite directions. That kind of elasticity not only makes styling a real joy, but also renders the hair resistant to fraying, splitting, and breaking.

By now, you've probably figured out what we're going to say next: There is no simple, long-lasting way to introduce new moisture into the keratin cells of a dried-out hair shaft. The trick, of course, is to retain natural moisture, which can be readily accomplished if you protect your hair from the dehydrating effects of overwashing, excessive blow-drying, strong chemical treatments, and prolonged UV exposure. Sun damage, incidentally, is an easily overlooked (yet very common!) source for many otherwise unexplainable bad hair days.

BASIC CARE I: HAIR WASHING

For most of us, washing the hair doesn't qualify as a top-of-mind experience. We do it, if not thoughtlessly, then at least mechanically. It's part of our daily routine, just like brushing our teeth, letting the dog out, or flipping through the morning paper. Conversely, special hair treatments such as perming, waving, tinting, or dyeing are usually given a measure of priority, probably because they are done less frequently, produce immediately visible results, and require a larger investment of time and money than mere hair washing.

If you truly care about the way your hair looks day in and day out, however, you would do well to reverse those priorities and devote more thought and energy to the seemingly mundane task of washing. Most women nowadays wash their hair on a daily basis, which means that the results, whether for good or ill, compound over time. When performed gently and correctly, washing can help you achieve clean, healthy hair that always has lots of life, lustre, and bounce. But when the job is done poorly or incorrectly, the damage just gets worse and worse, turning hair that ought to be perfectly manageable into an unruly mess that can't hold a set or even stand up to combing and brushing without splitting and breakage.

Choosing Your Shampoo

As with facial cleansing, washing the hair properly begins with selecting the right shampoo for your type of hair. In Chapter Two, *In Your Face! Cleansers & Cleansing for Best Results*, we recommended that you purchase the strongest facial cleanser you could find that would not irritate or dry out your skin. We feel pretty much the same way about shampoos, and advise that you opt for the most effective cleanser your hair can handle, but *stop short of any shampoo that irritates the scalp or leaves your hair feeling dry, coarse or brittle.* To be fair, we should tell you at this point that many well-respected dermatologists and hair care professionals put less emphasis on a shampoo's cleansing ability than we do, and more on mildness. These experts would encourage you to choose the gentlest available shampoo, provided it still managed to clean your hair. They would contend, with some justification, that the hair shaft is a fragile structure that should be protected from the oil-stripping action of a strong cleanser with shampoo additives[3] like proteins, vitamins, and moisturizers.

While we totally agree with all of this in theory, our real world experience has shown us that most women err on the side of buying shampoos that are milder than necessary. As a consequence, they wash their hair frequently—in most cases, at least five or more times per week—but it never feels quite clean to them because the shampoo they've chosen isn't strong enough to cut through the mixture of dust, grit, grease, and last night's hair spray that has accumulated since the previous mild washing. One ineffective cleansing follows another, and over time the combination of daily washing and daily blow-drying, and the build-up of residual shampoo particles renders the hair drier and more brittle than ever. In the user's mind, this only confirms her suspicion that she needs a mild, moisturizing shampoo for her exceptionally "dry" hair. But to our way of thinking, she might be smarter to use a stronger cleanser with less frequency, and thus give her hair and scalp the chance to recover and rehydrate between washings. A separately packaged conditioner, if needed, could then be used on "off" days should the hair show signs of dryness.

Now, this isn't to suggest that a very gentle shampoo can't be the right choice for you. If you currently use, say, a protein-enriched conditioning shampoo and it not only keeps your hair clean but also helps mend split ends and brings a little volume to the party, so much the better. Some people do possess naturally dry hair or limp hair that lacks body, in which case a mild, conditioning shampoo makes perfect sense. But what must be understood is that mildness can only be achieved by sacrificing a certain amount of cleansing power.[4] That's the way it works with bar soaps, and with shampoos as well. The critical item is to determine where your shampoo ought to fall in the broad range of options between the strongest detergent and dandruff-fighting shampoos on the one hand, and the mildest moisturizing and conditioning shampoos on the other.

Types of Shampoo

On a very basic level, there are two types of shampoos: cleansing shampoos and conditioning shampoos. Cleansing shampoos are designed to dissolve dirt, oil, and other impurities from the hair shaft with a high degree of efficiency; conditioning shampoos contain special additives that are intended to improve the appearance of your hair and make it easier to style. Both types of shampoo, significantly, also contain softening ingredients that counteract the degreasing effect of the cleansers used in the product. Cleansing shampoos such as Prell and Breck simply lack the cosmetic and styling additives found in conditioning shampoos. Of course, when you walk into your corner drugstore, you won't see anything nearly so clear-cut and uncomplicated as the tidy little division we've described here. What you will see, if you look at all closely, is a remarkable array of products created for an equally remarkable array of practical and aesthetic purposes.

Sure, one bottle of shampoo may seem to be nothing more than an amber version of the green bottle sitting next to it on the shelf. But in this instance, appearances can definitely be deceiving. An individual bottle of shampoo may contain upward of twenty different ingredients, some of which are included for cleansing, others for lathering, others for conditioning, and still others for moisturizing, stabilization,[5] product color, scent and so forth. Formulas, even for fairly "simple" shampoos, are exceedingly complex, and the results a given shampoo can be expected to produce will depend not only on the ingredients used by the manufacturer but also on the relative strength of each ingredient in the formulation. As a result, two bottles of shampoo with lists of ingredients that match up almost one to one can behave quite differently on your head because they were blended differently.

To give a somewhat oversimplified analogy, consider what

would happen if you were handed two recipes for chocolate chip cookies, both of which called for the use of salt and sugar, among other things. If the ratio of salt to sugar was one part salt to five parts sugar in the first recipe, but the reverse in the second (or even one part salt to three parts sugar), the two sets of cookies would not taste very much alike after you baked them. Now, imagine the number of variations possible when a gifted chemist has some fifteen, twenty or more ingredients at his or her disposal, all of which interact with one another in different ways depending on the relative strength in the formula. As you might have guessed, the possibilities are virtually endless. On the downside, this makes reading and truly understanding the list of ingredients on a shampoo bottle practically impossible for even the most knowledgeable consumer. The stuff is just too complex. On the plus side, all that mixing and blending of ingredients typically serves an important purpose: to create a shampoo that strikes some sort of balance between cleansing and conditioning. Certain shampoos will emphasize one quality or the other, but nearly every product on the market today strives to do at least a little of both.

When people ask us how to tell shampoos apart, we often suggest that they read the *front* of the bottle rather than the back. Generally speaking, manufacturers are not one bit shy about promoting the special properties of their various shampoos, and will also try to call your attention to any important additives they've included in their formulas. To help you sort through the various claims you'll encounter, it's worthwhile to review a short list of the most common terms used on shampoo bottles and in advertisements for shampoos. Some of these terms are general ("Conditioning shampoo"); others refer to a specific additive ("Contains antioxidant vitamins"). Let's take a look at the general terms first, but with the understanding that our list isn't even close to being exhaustive, since a really thorough examination of shampoo varieties and shampoo additives would require a book of its own. We'll start with the most broad-based term on our list, conditioning shampoos, then move on to terms that describe specific types of conditioning shampoos, and last, to a few of the more popular shampoo additives.

Conditioning shampoos, as you can gather from the term, are formulated to both cleanse your hair and serve as a conditioner. Like a conditioner, these products are designed to produce a variety of aesthetic results, including softening the hair, thickening the hair, improving manageability, adding sheen, and repairing split ends. Of course, not every conditioning shampoo will accomplish each of these fine things for you, but most will do more than one. We consumers, by the way, seem to appreciate the convenience of having our shampoo and conditioner in a single container, as evidenced by the fact that conditioning shampoos outnumber and outsell traditional cleansing shampoos by a wide margin.

This widespread popularity, however, does not necessarily equate with superior performance for every hair type: People with normal hair, oily hair or dandruff, for example, may find it advisable to try something stronger, while those of us with hair that tangles badly or splits easily may wish to use a separately packaged conditioner as a supplement to our conditioning shampoo. In the end, the suitability of a given product for your hair type will depend mainly on the shampoo's attributes (softens, adds sheen, etc.) and your specific needs (to build body, add lustre, etc.).

Protein-enriched shampoos constitute a special category of conditioning shampoos, and are formulated to improve the appearance of damaged hair. The protein in these shampoos, which may appear in the product as any one of a number of different additives, not only coats damaged hair shafts but also fills in cracks and pitted areas, resulting in hair that looks fuller, thicker, and glossier. Proteins are utilized for this purpose because they bind well with the cuticle covering of the hair shaft, which itself is a structural protein. Protein-enriched shampoos are particularly well suited for use on hair that has been damaged by dyes, waves, straighteners, and other chemical processes.

Balsam, a natural resin, has a well-established track record as a shampoo additive that strengthens and thickens the hair by restoring rigidity to damaged hair shafts. It is often paired with protein additives in body-building shampoos. In such formulations, balsam repairs the shaft from the inside, while the proteins go to work on the outside.

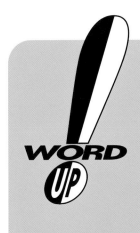

WORD UP

When your once lovely locks have been taxed to the max by harsh chemical treatments like dyeing and waving, the result is *processed hair.* And believe us, it's not a pretty sight! Processed hair is hair that looks like hay—dull, dry, lifeless, and prone to splitting and breakage.

To avoid it: Don't overprocess your hair; use chemical treatments sparingly. Also, give the hair some time to rest and rehydrate between chemical treatments, and never, ever apply more than one chemical treatment to your hair on the same day—or even on consecutive days, if you can help it.

To cure it: Cut the chemicals from your hair care regimen immediately, then go chemical-free for at least a week or two so that healthy new growth can replace damaged old growth. While you're waiting for that new growth to emerge, rehydrate and repair your processed hair with a protein-rich, moisturizing shampoo or conditioner.

Moisturizing shampoos comprise yet another category of conditioning shampoo. As the term implies, these shampoos are designed to help the hair retain vital moisture and oils. In fact, they often contain ingredients identical to those used in skin moisturizers, such as soy lecithin and lactic acid. A moisturizing shampoo is usually a good choice for anyone with naturally dry hair or for folks who spend lots of time outdoors, where the wind and sun combine to strip hair of the lubrication needed to keep it soft and manageable. For obvious reasons, moisturizing shampoos are typically a poor choice for those of us with oily or limp hair.

Herbal ingredients are now included in a large (and growing!) number of shampoos, supposedly for their ability to soften the hair and intensify its color. But while many herbs deliver these benefits in their natural state, none that we know of do so as shampoo additives. The reason for this ineffectiveness is twofold: First, the concentration of herbal ingredients in most shampoos is so low that the herbs might as well have been left out from the beginning; and second, the manufacturing process completely dilutes whatever softening or color-enhancing properties the herbs may have once had—just as it does with the herbal ingredients found in some bar soaps.

Aloe, which is derived from the succulent plant of the same name, has become a fairly popular shampoo additive over the years, perhaps because it is so well recognized by consumers for its capacity to soothe sunburn and ward off those pesky insects that bother us at the beach. Research, however, suggests that it doesn't possess any special properties that are beneficial to the hair.

Honey, like aloe, is another common additive that appeals to the ever-growing market for "natural" ingredients, yet doesn't have any real impact on a shampoo's ability to cleanse or condition the hair. What's more, honey is water-soluble, so any potential positive effect it might have gets washed down the drain with your shampoo lather.

Vitamins, especially those that fall into the anti-oxidant group, have long been used with some success in topical skin medications such as Retin-A™. But as shampoo additives, they have largely disappointed. The one notable exception to this rule is vitamin B_5, which you will find named as either panthenol or pantyl in a list of ingredients. Unlike other vitamins used in shampoos, vitamin B_5 in its chemical form has the ability to penetrate the hair shaft and strengthen the strand from the inside out. Not surprisingly, it is often added as a conditioning agent in body-building shampoos.

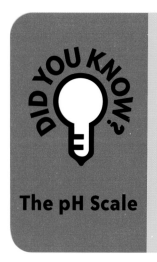

DID YOU KNOW?

The pH Scale

The *pH scale* is used to gauge the degree of acidity or alkalinity in many different kinds of substances, including hair care products. The scale runs from 0 to 14, with zero being completely acid and 14, completely alkaline.[6] Shampoos and conditioners, on the whole, tend to be alkaline (or high pH), which can be stressful to dry or damaged hair. *pH-balanced* or *low pH* products are therefore often recommended for hair that is dehydrated, overprocessed, or brittle. A shampoo or conditioner with a pH of 7 is considered balanced, and anything below 7 is considered a low pH product.

Sunscreen ingredients such as cinnamates and PABA are found not only in products designed for the skin, but in many shampoos as well. These shampoos provide useful protection against UV radiation to your hair and, to a lesser extent, your scalp, but do nothing to reduce the hair damage caused by heat and dehydration. So, while a shampoo that contains sunscreen additives is preferable to one that offers no UV protection at all, your hair—and, more important, your face—will find much safer shelter beneath a broad-brimmed, tightly woven hat.

JUST YOUR TYPE!

Now that you know a little bit about the various types of shampoos and the additives commonly used in them, the logical question to ask is: "What's right for me?" But as you might have guessed, we cannot provide a "one size fits all" solution. Hair types and hair problems vary from one person to the next, and need to be considered when choosing a shampoo. Fortunately, most modern shampoos are gentle enough that any error you might commit, aside from washing too often, won't result in utter disaster. As a starting point, consult the guidelines below to match your hair type with a shampoo type. Then, once you've selected the general type of shampoo you want (low pH, cleansing, etc.), narrow your search by identifying any special needs or problems you have and looking for a product that contains additives that specifically address them.

Try low pH or pH-balanced shampoos for…
- Dry, brittle hair
- Processed hair
- Sun damaged hair

Try cleansing shampoos for…
- Oily hair
- Normal, trouble-free hair

Try body-building shampoos for…
- Limp hair
- Thin hair
- Hair that covers poorly

Try baby shampoo for…
- Exceptionally thin, wispy hair

Determining Your Hair Type

The terms people use to describe the major hair types are almost identical to those applied to skin types: oily, dry, and normal. The similarity isn't accidental, either. An individual's hair type and skin type are usually closely matched, meaning that if you have, say, an oily complexion, your hair probably tends to be oily, too. Exceptions, of course, can and do occur. But the general rule is accurate more often than not. This correlation exists because both the face and the scalp rely on the sebaceous (or oil) glands not only to supply moisture, but to help retain it as well. The scalp, in fact, is merely a continuation of the skin of the face, so it stands to reason that the oil glands there operate in a manner similar to that of the glands that control sebum production on nearby facial regions.

Dry Hair

Naturally dry hair, like naturally dry skin, is relatively rare in teens. As we've seen, most young people possess very productive oil glands as a result of the heightened hormonal activity that occurs during this stage of life. When a teen has dry hair, then, the cause is more often external than internal, and usually stems from overuse of hair styling chemicals, excessive blow-drying, washing too frequently, too much sun, or any combination of the above. But since a small percentage of teens do have naturally dry hair, it's helpful to know how to spot the difference between hair that was "born" dry and hair that has been "worn" dry.

The strength of the hair shaft is the best means of determining the difference. Now, any hair shaft that is dry will tend to be somewhat stiff and dull looking, owing to its lack of moisture. But a naturally dry hair shaft will retain its strength and resist snapping when combed or brushed, while a hair shaft that has been dried out by processing or UV exposure will almost always be brittle and susceptible to breakage. Some other indicators of naturally dry hair are:

- dry complexion
- sensitive scalp
- hair that requires washing just once or twice a week
- hair that holds a set well and styles easily

- hands that chap easily and require frequent use of moisturizers
- dark, thick, curly hair
- hair that is easily damaged by processing or UV exposure
- "dry scalp" dandruff

Oily Hair

Oily hair, no surprise, is much more common among teens than dry hair is, again as a result of the perfectly natural hormonal activity tied to growth and development. Oily hair typically exhibits a nice, vibrant sheen—especially after washing—and stands up well to processing. However, it also requires frequent cleansing and probably doesn't hold a set or retain styling as long as you'd like. Among the signs of hair that is oilier than normal, we may include:

- oily complexion
- acne-prone skin
- need for frequent hair washing
- hair that looks slick and feels greasy when not washed for a day or two
- hair that resists styling and wants to cling to the scalp
- presence of dandruff, though this widespread disorder can occur with all hair types

A SIMPLE, EFFECTIVE HAIR WASHING REGIMEN

OK. You know your hair type and you've chosen a shampoo that suits it. The shampoo cleanses well enough that you probably don't need to wash your hair every day, and perhaps contains conditioning ingredients designed to help handle one or two problems you commonly encounter. Now you're ready to head to the shower and shampoo effectively, yet gently. Here's how, in four quick steps.

Step 1: Pre-rinse. Soak your hair thoroughly, craning your head forward so that the water runs from back to front. If you have relatively long hair, gather it up and flip it forward to ensure a good rinse. You may find that the entire process is easier if you *stand with your back to the shower head as opposed to facing it.* This will almost surely feel awkward at first, since most folks like to tilt their face up toward the shower head and let the water run from the top of the forehead back. But that's precisely what we want you to avoid. The strands along the edge of your forehead and at the sides of your hairline are typically the shortest and most brittle on your scalp. When you subject them to intense water pressure, you encourage split ends and breakage. Rinsing from back to front allows you to avoid this problem. Another advantage of the back-to-front rinse is that it virtually guarantees that the roots will be as well rinsed and well cleansed as the ends, an especially important consideration for anyone prone to dandruff or scaling of the scalp.

Finally, adjust the water temperature of your rinse to suit your hair type. Coarse or unruly hair generally responds best to warmer water, while fine, limp hair usually likes a lukewarm rinse. The reason: The curls and kinks in coarse hair require hot water to help break down the strong hydrogen bonds that caused the strands to bend this way and that in the first place. Limp hair, conversely, needs all the body it can get, so you don't want to further weaken its already frail molecular bonds with water that's too hot.

Step 2: Applying shampoo. Pour enough shampoo into the palm of your hand to lather your hair deeply and completely. The amount of shampoo required will vary depending on the density of the product's concentration (i.e., how much or how little water the formula contains), as well as the length and thickness of your hair. A full tablespoon, give or take, should be about the right quantity in most cases. Next, gently work the shampoo into your hair, using a massaging motion with the tips of your fingers. Take your time and make sure the shampoo lather penetrates down to the roots and scalp. If you cover these areas well, the ends will take care of themselves. Also, be attentive to the hair around your temples and along the nape of your neck. These spots are often glossed over too lightly or, even worse, missed entirely.

Step back from the water while you apply the shampoo, and allow the lather to stand for 30 to 60 seconds before rinsing it out. This gives the shampoo adequate time to bind chemically with the hair shafts. If you rinse too hastily, you'll be removing the shampoo from your hair before it has a chance to do its job.

Step 3: Cleansing rinse. Rinse under cool or tepid water until every trace of shampoo has been removed from your hair, again with your back to the onrushing water and your head craned forward. A complete cleansing rinse will probably take more time than you think—a full minute at a minimum, and somewhat longer if your hair is at all thick or bushy. If you like, you can speed up the process a bit by massaging your hair during the rinse.

Step 4: Drying. First blot excess moisture from your hair with a thick, absorbent bath towel, then comb while the hair is still fairly wet. If you towel-dry your hair, be sure to use a blotting or patting motion, as opposed to a vigorous rubbing that can lead to fraying and breakage. If you blow-dry your hair, do so at a moderate heat setting, following the guidelines set forth below.

Washing Your Hair: How Often Is Too Often?

As recently as the 1960s, most people washed their hair just once a week, or twice a week, tops. Styles back then were shorter, and the cleansers people used on their hair were by and large stronger. But today, daily washing is the accepted standard, especially in the U.S. This increase in the number of weekly washings has been made possible by—and gained momentum from—the rapid and continuing development of gentler shampoos and more effective conditioners, as well as our national preoccupation with personal hygiene and cleanliness. Many shampoos, in fact, are now formulated with the idea of daily usage in mind. However, unless your scalp and hair are very oily or you work in an exceptionally grimy environment, once a day is probably more washing than your hair really needs. If you find that your scalp and hair are prone to dryness, but your complexion isn't, you should try keeping the cap on that shampoo bottle for a day or two, just as a test. It could be that the problem isn't the lack of natural moisture in your hair, but how often you wash it.

BASIC CARE II: BLOW-DRYING

The logical consequence of daily hair washing is, of course, daily hair drying, which most people nowadays accomplish with the aid of an electric blow-dryer. Blow-drying is not only a quick and easy means of drying even the fullest head of hair, but in the right hands serves as a marvelous styling tool as well. In addition, blow-drying—if done correctly—can be less taxing to the hair than old-fashioned towel-drying: You're unlikely, for example, to accidentally snap and fray strands along the hairline with a blow-dryer the way you can when rubbing forcefully with a towel.

The most common problem with blow-drying, in fact, isn't the blow-dryer, but the person holding the handle. Too often, she's either in a huge rush to get her hair dried fast, and so operates the machine at its maximum power setting; or she absolutely refuses to leave the house with even slightly damp hair, and so runs the device until every last root is not just dry but positively parched. The outcome in both instances is the same: The hair becomes extremely dry and brittle because it's constantly being stripped of the natural hydrolipidic film (a mixture of sebum and water) that helps keep it soft and supple under ordinary circumstances. As the overdrying continues, split ends develop, lustre is diminished, and moisture-starved hairs weaken to the point that they snap at the touch of a comb.

The obvious solution is to blow your hair dry, not blow it away. Set your dryer on low or moderate heat, never high, and dry the hair in sections, lifting gently to expose the roots as you go. Work slowly and methodically, but keep it moving. If you linger on any one spot long enough to make your hair or scalp feel hot to the touch, you've overstayed your welcome. Stop when the hair *looks* dry, but still feels a tad damp, especially at the roots. Then let the air finish the job while you dress and have breakfast. Last, if you use mousse, gel, or hair spray, wait until your hair has air-dried completely before applying them. Most hair styling products won't bind as well to a slightly moist hair strand as they will to one that has dried fully.

BASIC CARE III: BRUSHING & COMBING

When you brush and/or comb your hair, you do more than just style it. You also clean it by removing loose particles like those left behind by old shampoo and conditioner; nourish it by descaling and stimulating the scalp, which improves circulation and brings more oxygen and nutrient-rich blood to your hair roots; and add to the impression of volume by gently lifting hair strands away from the scalp. To that extent, combing and brushing are important yet easily overlooked components of any hair care regimen. Proper brushing and combing is a simple matter, and can be covered with a few basic dos and don'ts.

The dos:

- Do choose combs and brushes that are soft and flexible (see below for details).
- Do brush your hair at least once a day, but not more than twice, starting underneath at the scalp and working out to the ends. Also, brush from the back forward—not from the top back—to help prevent split ends.
- Do comb with a light touch, adding a dab of moisturizer or cream rinse conditioner to the comb's teeth if you find that it wants to grab and snag.

The don'ts:

- Don't ever yank or jerk your way through a snag; the reason it hurts is because you're literally tearing out your hair.
- Don't become obsessive about brushing or combing. Too much of either damages the cuticle covering of your hair strands, resulting in split ends, broken hairs, and diminished lustre.
- Don't stick with a cut or style—even one you like a lot—that necessitates constant brushing and combing. You'll wind up doing more harm to your hair than the style is worth.

How To Prevent That Light-Socket Look

If you have too much static electricity in your hair or fly-away hair, the typical response is to reach for a bottle of hair spray. An easier solution—and one that's less taxing to your hair—is to lightly spritz your hair brush with cling-free spray, which can be found at just about any drugstore or supermarket. This will serve to neutralize static build-up and help keep those over-charged hairs where they belong.

Choosing a Comb That Won't Take a Bite Out of Your Hair

We've just seen that combing too often—or too vigorously—can fray and break your hair. And so, too, can your choice of comb. The hair breakers? Combs with stiff, tightly bunched teeth and sharp, pointed tips, which are a definite "don't" for most folks, but especially for those of us with really long hair or dry, brittle, split-prone hair. Instead, look for a comb with widely spaced, flexible teeth and soft, rounded tips. To test, simply press the comb you own—or want to buy—teeth down into the palm of your hand. A comb that feels stiff and sharp probably (who'da thunk it?) *is* stiff and sharp, while a more forgiving comb will bend easily under moderate pressure and leave just a modest impression on your palm.

The same principles apply to brushes, too. Here again, you want softness and flexibility for fewer broken hairs and split ends. Soft-bristled brushes come in two basic varieties: those made from natural fibers such as animal hair, and those made of very pliable synthetic materials with rounded rubber tips. Brushes with natural-fiber bristles are generally the least damaging to your hair, but either kind is preferable to a stiff nylon brush with razor-sharp tips.

An exception: People with very thick or curly hair may discover to their dismay that a flexible, soft-bristled brush simply cannot flow smoothly through their tangled locks. If this is the case for you, look for a moderately stiff brush or comb before resorting to the stiffest one you can find. The stiffer model may seem easier to use, but only because it's ripping (as opposed to running) through your hair.

100 Strokes . . .

with a wet noodle to anyone out there who persists in believing that ceaseless combing and brushing are good ways to "train" the hair to lay properly. *Please note:* Your hair should never be "trained," "tamed," or disciplined in any manner—even when it behaves quite badly. Get a cut that complements the natural texture and growth patterns of your hair, and you will soon find that it lays beautifully and styles easily with *less* combing and brushing, not more.

Tender, Loving Care: Scalp Massage

Scalp massage delivers many of the benefits of brushing, but to a higher degree and with less stress to your hair. These benefits include the loosening of scales from the scalp, better circulation, and improved flow of oil from the sebaceous glands of the scalp to the hair shafts. Scalp massage is also faster than brushing. The warm, tingly feeling that tells you the small blood vessels of the scalp have been thoroughly stimulated usually occurs after just a few minutes of massage, as opposed to 10 minutes or more for brushing. Plus, you don't run nearly as much risk of fraying hairs and splitting ends with massage.

To stimulate your scalp manually, simply use the padded part of your fingertips to gently massage every portion of the scalp. Work with both hands at once; exert steady, even pressure; and massage in a circular motion, concentrating on only a small section of the scalp at a time. Once the area being massaged feels warm and tingly, move on to the next spot. We like to start at the crown, advance to the forehead, then make our way down the sides to finish at the back of the head and neck. You can follow our routine, or try your own. The important thing is to have a system that ensures thorough coverage of the entire scalp.

One word of warning: If your hair and scalp tend to be very oily, you should probably consider using an electric scalp vibrator rather than your hands when you massage. The oils from your fingertips and hands can intensify the oiliness of your hair and thus aggravate your problem. Electric scalp massagers are available at most stores that sell other hair care appliances such as blow-dryers and curling irons.

CREATIVE CARE: STYLING TIPS

Great looking locks are the end result of intelligent daily care and savvy styling. Care comes first, because you simply cannot properly style hair that lacks natural body, lustre, and manageability, which is why we've devoted so much of our discussion thus far to the basics of everyday maintenance. Hopefully, the guidelines we've laid down will help you establish a regimen that keeps your hair clean and strong, yet soft and nicely lubricated too. Once you reach that point, you're ready to optimize the appearance of your healthy head of hair through creative styling. This is the fun, artistic part of hair care—your chance to go for the looks you've always wanted but perhaps couldn't carry off before because you either lacked the know-how or because your hair wasn't healthy enough to cooperate. We'll cover several different looks, with an emphasis on those that require more than mere brushing and combing to achieve. Along the way, we'll share stylists' secrets that will not only make the job easier but also add those finishing touches that can transform an ordinary "do" into something really special.

Choosing a Style You Can Live With

Sometimes the gap between the look you want and a look that you can realistically maintain can be too wide. If your typical weekday, for instance, consists of exercise in the morning, then school, then band practice, then dinner, then homework, then sleep, chances are you won't be able to carry off some of the more labor-intensive styles you saw in the most recent issue of *Glamour*. This isn't to suggest that you aren't attractive enough to wear your hair that way or that you don't possess the savvy and energy to make it work. But the fact is that most busy teens simply don't have the time needed to do all the curling, teasing, spritzing, brushing, and blow-drying it takes to support an extravagantly coiffed head of hair.

Below:

Select a style you can live with and one that looks great on you. Kris found that a shorter cut works best for her.

If you happen to have the time, then great. You'll find plenty of helpful tips in the following section of this chapter. But if not, you're probably better off adopting a more practical approach

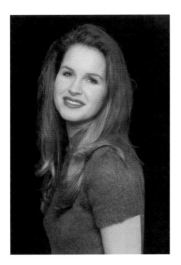
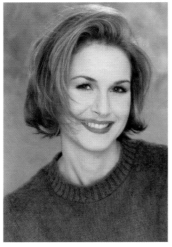
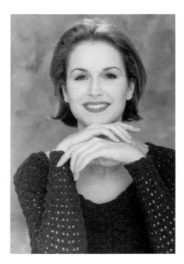

and matching your hairstyle to your lifestyle. Shorter cuts, of course, are easiest to maintain, as are styles that accentuate the natural qualities of your hair. If you have a stylist you know and trust, set aside 15 or 20 minutes to talk with her or him about your hair and the types of cuts that will allow it to grow out naturally without a lot of primping and preening. Our guess is that you'll not only save time every day for having done so, but also wind up looking better than ever.

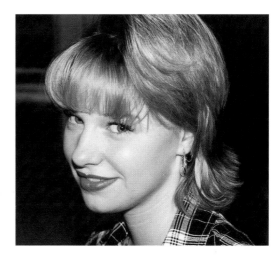

Variations on the Layered Look

If texture is what you're looking for, get a cut with plenty of layers built in to add movement (think Courteney Cox) but no blunt lines. To break up straight lines, work a texturizing styling gel (Salon Selectives Kiwi Jasmine Texturizing Gel or L'Oreal Studio Line Mega Gel) or a leave-in conditioner (like Aussie Dew Plex) through damp hair, then blow-dry. While blow-drying, use your fingers as a brush, tousling your hair at the roots. When your hair is dry, put a bit more gel on your fingers and separate out some pieces around your face, ears, etc. If your hair is medium to thick, try shampooing every other day for a messier, more tousled look. If added volume is what you want—fluffy, puffy, supermodel-y locks, the hair equivalent of a down jacket—leave the cap on the conditioner and blow-dry after washing, with your head forward, drying from back to front.

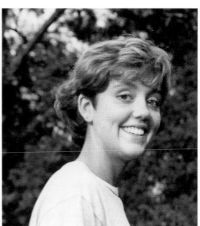

Above:
Layered cuts are great for adding texture and volume.

Fuller Looks for Limp Locks

Good news: Your limp locks can be cured, at least temporarily, with dozens of products designed to deliver the fullness required for certain styles. Unfortunately, many products with similar sounding names are not at all alike. Results can vary widely from one item (or brand) to the next, and the success of a given product depends greatly on whether it's appropriate for the styling method you've chosen. To help you sort through your choices,

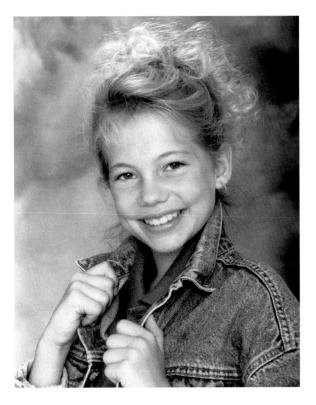

Above:
Styling products such as gels, mousses, & texturizers produce lots of volume.

we'll play matchmaker here, and marry a few popular styles to the volumizing goods you'll need to attain them.

For the kind of bouncy, high-energy waves that look great against your shoulders as you walk down the street, choose a body-building mousse like Salon Selectives Bodifying Mousse or L'Oreal Studio Line Mega Mousse. To apply, simply comb in through damp, towel-dried hair from roots to tips. For maximum effect, try this stylist's trick: Divide the hair on each side of your head into eight small sections—four in a horizontal row just in front of your crown, and four directly behind. Then, set damp hair on large velcro rollers.

For a tousled—yet still full—look, choose texturizing or thickening sprays like Paul Mitchell Volumizing Spray or Aveda Purescriptions Volumizing Finisher. To apply, towel-dry your hair, then direct spray at roots and at any spots where you want added volume. For a tousled look with even more volume, blow-dry rather than towel-dry, bending forward as you do so and fluffing the hair at the roots with your fingertips. Spritz on volumizing spray a few times while you dry, then finish with conventional hairspray to keep the whole affair from collapsing.

Another way to add fullness is to shampoo your roots really well with a body-building shampoo such as Vidal Sassoon Shampoo A Extra or Revlon Outrageous Volumizing Shampoo. Be careful, though, to avoid overuse of these protein-rich formulations, especially if you also use lots of special gels and mousses. If that's the case, put the fancy stuff away at least once a week and lather up with a deep-cleansing shampoo to remove volume-killing product build-up. Along the same lines, if you need a conditioner for detangling, choose a superlight rinse-out variety (such as Aussie Slip Detangler or Joico Lite Instant

Detangler & Conditioner), and apply it only to the ends. For overall volume, work in a body-boosting gel mousse like Regis Dual Action Gel-Mousse or Dep Extra Body Mousse 'N Gel, both of which enhance fullness and improve control.

For a lift at the roots, try a volumizing spray or gel. Aveda Volumizing Tonic is a good example of the former, Dep Root Boost of the latter. After applying either of these products, turn your head upside down and blow-dry, lifting hair away from your head and rubbing the roots with your fingertips. When your hair is almost dry, flip your head back up and blow-dry your hair section by section with a jumbo round brush, pulling the brush the opposite direction of your hair's natural growth pattern. A stylist secret for max lift: Roll up a few sections at the crown with large velcro rollers when your hair is dry. Heat with a blow-dryer for 10 minutes, allow to cool for another 10 minutes, then unwind rollers and fluff hair with your fingers.

If you want smooth body, use a volumizing shampoo like Bare Essentuals Full Body Shampoo or J.F. Lazartique Body-Giving Shampoo, followed by a volumizing tonic or "serum" like Redken Fat Cat Volumist or Systeme Biolage Daily Leave-In Tonic. After shampooing, simply use your hands to distribute the tonic through towel-dried hair from roots to tips, then blow-dry with a large round brush, grasping sections of hair by the roots and curving them under as you go.

Finally, to keep your new "do" from falling flat, try Vidal Sassoon Extra Body Mousse. This is a product we like a lot because it provides the kind of volume everyone hopes for, but without weighing down the hair. To apply it, first work the mousse through damp hair, concentrating on the roots. Next, lift the hair away from the roots while blow-drying, then remove heat and continue holding hair until it cools and sets.

Frizz & Curl Control

If you'd like to sport springy, shiny, spirally curls like Nicole Kidman's or Julia Roberts', but have a frizzy mess to cope with instead, there are several things you can do to regain control and restore some semblance of style. For starters, recall that frizzy hair tends to be dry hair, so load up on conditioner in the shower, using a wide-tooth comb to distribute it through the hair, then rinse. If your hair is super dry and coarse, try leaving in a bit of conditioner—enough that your hair feels slippery to the touch even after the rinse. Next, you need to select the right styling product: For tight, frizzy curls, go for a curl-controlling mousse (Clairol Frizz Control Restructurizing Mousse) or gel (L'Oreal Studio Line Lasting Curls or Vavoom Smoothing Gel). For wavy hair that turns wiry when the humidity rises, try a frizz-busting leave-in conditioner like Clairol Frizz Control Taming Balm. Don't brush or comb after application. Instead, separate and shape the curls with your fingers. Let your hair air dry, or blow-dry with a diffuser attachment. Want to know what the stylists do for photo-shoot-perfect results? Then try these tips: Refine the curls around your face with a curling iron when the hair is dry; or set damp hair in jumbo pin curls, then blow-dry with a diffuser and allow to cool before unwinding. Either method, done carefully and correctly, should yield curls you can be proud of.

It's also important to pamper your dry, frizzy locks with nourishing moisturizers, such as Ouidad Deep Conditioner, a lotion for frizzy, curly hair that has drawn raves from beauty editors across the country. Ouidad's New York City salon, in fact, has evolved into something of a mecca for the curly-headed crowd. And while you may not be able to afford to fly there and schedule an appointment, this top stylist does offer a full selection of hair care products that are available to anyone, anywhere. For a free brochure of Ouidad's complete line, call the salon toll-free at 1-800-677-HAIR, visit their web site at www.ouidad.com (code W9709), or write to Ouidad, PO Box 80, Bethel, CT 06801.

Fashion Tool Box: Curl Control

To get the curls you want, owning the right appliances and implements is an absolute must. Here's a short list of useful tools, with notes on the styles they can help you achieve.

For loose waves, we recommend a blow-dryer-and-round-brush-in-one, which is designed to be used on damp hair. This device helps lift the roots on cropped cuts, and imparts gently flowing waves to hair that's chin-length or longer. Just brush through from the roots, curving the ends in the direction you want the waves to go. Conair's Big Curls Hot Air Brush is ideal for this kind of loose-wave styling.

For big, bodaciously bouncy curls, try hot rollers with easy-to-use clips that shape full curls with plenty of body. The key here is to roll toward the roots so you don't wind up with ridges in your curls. Our tool of choice for big-curl girls: Revlon's Ultra Setter.

For precise ringlets, a curling iron with a small ½- to ¾-inch barrel and heat guard can work like a magic wand. Remington's Curl Styler is the one we like best, because it's positively perfect for creating corkscrews in medium to long hair. To style your hair this way, simply start at the root and wrap small sections of hair tightly around the iron all the way to the ends, then let the tool take over from there.

Playing It Straight

From what we can tell, there are two types of people in the world: those with straight hair who want curls; and those with curly hair they'd like to straighten. Since we've already addressed the styling dilemmas of limp, volume-challenged hair, it's time now to discuss how one can safely reduce waviness for straighter hair. Now, much has been said and written about the damage caused by chemical hair straighteners—and most of it is absolutely true! When you use a straightener—or nearly any chemical process—on your hair incorrectly or too frequently, you're begging for trouble. However, we also believe that periodic chemical straightening, particularly if it is done by an experienced stylist, is less harmful than applying direct heat from an iron every day.

If you feel you must straighten your hair, then, our first piece of advice is to have a qualified professional do it for you. Forget the at-home kits. Forget your friend's sister who "does this all

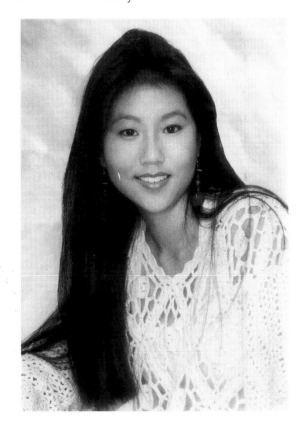

Below:
Long, sleek looks such as this can be achieved with a blow-dryer and the right styling products.

the time." Go to a pro, and get it done right so that your hair is less stressed and easier to style afterward. Also, take steps to improve the condition of your processed hair. Shampoo less frequently, using a low pH formulation, and apply a deep, protein-rich conditioner at least once a week. When your waves or curls start to reassert themselves, don't react immediately by running to the salon for another straightening. Instead, space your visits and use a blow-dryer to maintain the look in the meantime. To straighten with a blow-dryer, set the device at low or moderate heat and slowly dry your hair section by section with the aid of a round brush. Aim the dryer at the roots first, then work your way down to the ends, curling them under as you progress. Unroll each section gently, and continue until all sections are dry. Finish with a frizz-fighting pomade like Aveda Purefume Brilliante Humectant Pomade, Regis Shining Pomade, or KMS Pomade.

Is Your Hair Fit To Be Tied?

Corn rows, braids, ponytails, and other popular styles that contort your locks into unnatural positions can distress hair to (and past!) the breaking point. Lots of split ends and broken strands, especially along the hairline, indicate that you need to reduce wear and tear sooner rather than later. Here are a few simple tips that can help you minimize the damage:

Below:

Corn rows are a great-looking style that works equally well whether you are playing volleyball or dressing up for the prom.

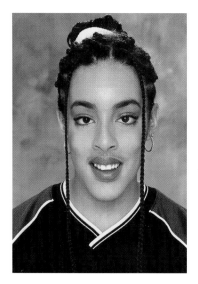

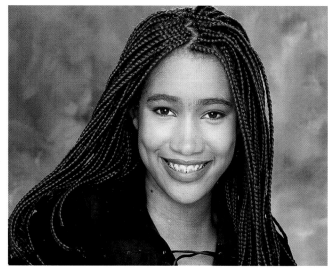

- Give your hair a chance to go its own way from time to time by periodically switching to a more natural style. Your friends will still recognize you, and your newly liberated hair will get a much-needed opportunity to relax, recover and regrow.
- Loosen up a little: Hair that's pulled too taut can be a real headache . . . and we mean that literally! To save yourself the discomfort and to avoid pulled-out strands, leave your hair loose around the roots when you tie or braid. Like to visualize? Think of gathering the hair, not pulling it.
- Ponytail holders are positively notorious for snagging hair, causing ends to split and strands to break. The slick solution: Grease your hairband with a dab of conditioner before you tie up.

How To Make Your Hair Do the Splits

If you'd like your hair to be dry as a bundle of dead twigs, and so split and frayed at the ends that you can't do a thing with it, we can offer several useful pointers. Follow *this* advice, and we promise you'll have hair that resembles the dangling remains of a broken tire-swing rope.

- Overuse plenty of harsh, moisture-sapping chemicals on a regular basis. Straighteners, bleaches, dyes, curling lotions, and permanent wave solutions will all serve nicely.
- Apply more than one of the above treatments to your hair on the same day.
- Leave just about any hair care product on your hair too long.
- Get compulsive about washing your hair. As you'll remember from Chapter Two, cleansing is an essentially drying, oil-sapping process. Shampooing too frequently is therefore a wonderful way to leave your hair bone dry.
- Blow-dry until it hurts. Put your machine on the highest setting, and let that sucker run. No one else in your house uses the bathroom, anyhow.
- Be really heavy-handed when you comb and brush to ensure that the strands you've weakened actually split,

fray, and break. Comb and brush often, at least several times a day.

- Give your hair some sun. It hasn't been out enough lately.

How To Keep Your Hair From Doing the Splits

We hope you laughed while reading the list above—it wasn't at all meant to be taken seriously. However, many people routinely commit nearly all of those blunders, mainly because they just don't know better. Proper hair care begins with understanding that your hair is part of the organ system known as the skin. And hair, like skin, loves the natural oils that keep it soft, smooth, and supple. (Where have you read those words before?) To keep your hair well lubed and looking sharp, kindly follow the real advice offered below.

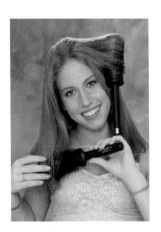

Above:
Styling tools can be your hair's best friend if used correctly.

- Pare your hair care arsenal down to the essentials, and use what's left as sparingly as possible. Harsh chemicals that make hair dry and brittle, such as bleaches and dyes, cause damage that can't be repaired except through cyclical regrowth, so lay off the rough stuff for a while when splitting, fraying, and breakage start to occur. While waiting for new hair to replace damaged hair, use a conditioner (or a conditioning shampoo) to make your hair *appear* softer and fuller.

- Never apply more than one chemical treatment to your hair on the same day. Also, if you bleach, dye, or tint, do your best to apply the product to new growth only. Applying it to old growth amounts to double-treating those strands, which fairly begs them to break.

- When using hair care products, always rinse them out thoroughly after the prescribed amount of time. Shampoo should also be rinsed completely from your hair. It's not uncommon for people to mistake dried particles of residual shampoo for dandruff flakes.

- Wash your hair only as often as necessary, using a shampoo that keeps it clean and manageable. If your hair is naturally dry, be especially wary of overwashing.

- If you blow-dry, do so at moderate heat, and stop before your hair dries completely. The ends should still be slightly damp to the touch when you're through with the machine.

- Comb and brush only as often as needed to keep yourself presentable, and use a light touch when you do. Overly vigorous combing and brushing are among the chief causes of damaged, broken hair. To stimulate the scalp, use massage in addition to your once-a-day brushing.
- Wear a hat to protect your hair (and scalp, and face!) whenever you'll be outside long enough to risk prolonged UV exposure.

HAIR TO DYE FOR

It's a fact: For as long as we human beings have walked the Earth, at least some percentage of us have wanted to change the color of our hair. This impulse is not only as strong as ever today, but also more easily gratified, thanks to advances in chemistry and the growth of the modern hair care industry. Dyes nowadays come in four basic varieties, which can be distinguished from one another by the permanence (or duration) of the color change they cause.

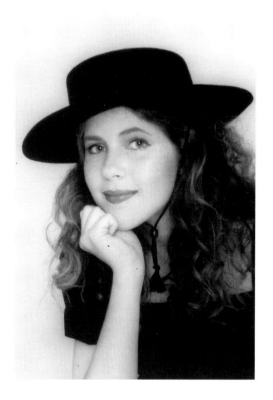

Above:
A hat can be a great accessory as well as protect your hair, scalp, and face from the sun.

1. **Temporary rinses** are designed for short-term use. The color they impart to your hair lasts only until your next hair washing.

2. **Gradual dyes** are specially formulated to help you avoid the appearance of an "overnight" change. These products change hair color over a period of 2 to 3 weeks.

3. **Semipermanent tints** create a color change that lasts through four to six hair washings, which means you will enjoy the new shade for as long as a month if you shampoo infrequently, or as little as a week if you wash your hair daily. Because semipermanent tints can only deposit color, they can be used to darken your hair but not lighten it. Many women who wish to lighten their hair temporarily do so by using bleach-based or peroxide-based treatments (Sun-In is a good example) that are designed to be sprayed on and combed in. These prod-

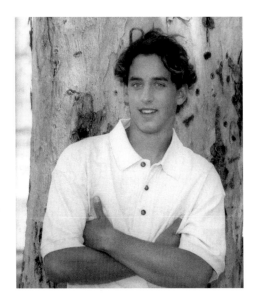

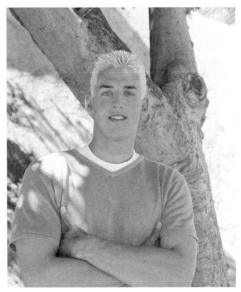

Above:

Experimenting with hair color allows you to try a whole new look.

ucts, though generally effective at lightening the hair, are also easily misapplied. Uneven application usually results in a blotchy look, and dark hair colors have a nasty tendency to turn orange, rather than, say, the soft brown envisioned by the user.

4. Permanent dyes don't wash out but aren't truly "permanent" in the strictest sense of the word, because they won't change the color of new growth. Even so, they last longer than any of the other options we've listed, especially if you color new growth as it comes in. When you touch up your hair with a permanent dye, you should try to apply the product to undyed areas only. This can be a somewhat tricky and time-consuming process, but it is more than worthwhile to be careful. Strands that get double-treated are likely to wind up in your brush or on the floor before their time.

Some General Guidelines

When it comes to hair dyeing, some folks opt for wholesale changes and splashy effects, while others wish only to tweak their natural shade or highlight certain aspects of it. But if you want a believable look—and it's perfectly acceptable if you don't, by the way—try to choose a shade that forms a natural combination with the color of your complexion and eyebrows. You won't see too many olive-skinned beauties, after all, sashaying about with naturally blonde hair, or many red-headed babies with jet-black eyebrows. Along a similar vein, it's usually best, at least initially, to go a shade lighter than the desired effect when darkening your hair, or a shade darker than you really want when lightening your hair. Granted, this is a conservative approach, but it will keep you from making a change that is more dramatic than you bargained for. Besides, if you don't care for the result, you'll still be closer to your natural color than if you had gone overboard, and you can always darken or lighten as necessary afterward. Go too wild, on the other hand, and you're often stuck until new growth pushes out the hairs you've dyed.

By and large, in fact, we like to see people stay within a shade of their natural color, at least at the outset. By starting with a subtle alteration of color, you greatly reduce the chances that you (not to mention your boyfriend, your classmates, and your co-workers) won't be shocked by what looks back at you from the bathroom mirror. At-home coloring mistakes can happen, especially when the person applying the process lacks experience in dyeing hair. However, minor adjustments can usually be made, *as long as you haven't strayed too far from your normal shade.* Let's run through a few examples of the most common errors, and suggest ways you can fix 'em should the need arise.

Problem: Your dyed hair is too blonde.

Solution: Recolor with a shade darker than the original dye, yet lighter than your natural color.

Problem: Your dyed hair isn't light enough.

Solution: A single process can only lighten dark brown hair so much. Try a double-process kit next time instead.

Problem: You've used a bleach-based dye on your hair, and now it's too brassy.

Solution: Bleach often has the tendency to redden hair, even though the color deposited by the dye is supposed to neutralize this effect. Next time around, try one of the natural dyes discussed in the following section of this chapter.

Problem: You've used dye to achieve a brunette color, but now find that your hair has an unattractive green cast to it.

Solution: It's likely you chose an ash-tone brunette color. Natural brown hair has red and gold tones, while ash is designed to neutralize those tones with a cool green or violet base. To lose the green, recolor with a warm red or golden brown.

Problem: You've dyed your light hair black in order to achieve a darker shade, but now it's going black . . . REALLY black.

Solution: Black isn't easily reversed, so you have only two options, neither of which is very appealing. One, wait for new growth to emerge and re-dye with dark brown. Two, go to a salon and have the color chemically removed.

Problem: You've dyed your hair red, and it's so brilliant people shade their eyes when you walk by.

Solution: Reds sometimes show up harshly on light hair. The quick fix is to tone it down for the time being with a semipermanent color in a cool natural or ash shade. Longer term, you'll want to use strawberry blonde and golden tints for a softer, more natural look.

Of course, the bizarre colors that result from dyes gone wrong come in every shade under the sun—as well as a few that have *never* seen the natural light of day. The mistakes we've just covered are merely a sampling of the ones we run across most often. When your at-home coloring presents you with a problem that you haven't the faintest idea how to solve, for gosh sakes, don't guess at a solution or attempt to fix it through trial and error. Visit a salon you trust and ask what can be done. Then pray the answer doesn't involve a pair of scissors!

It's Getting Thick Now!

Remember that dyes serve to thicken your hair by swelling the interior of the shaft and coating its cuticle covering. If you have thin hair, you'll probably consider this a blessing. But if your hair is already coarser and thicker than you'd like it to be, you may want to decide whether the color change is worth the added volume.

Henna & Other Natural Hair Care Products

Not every useful hair care product is packaged in a bottle. Some actually do grow on trees! As we noted earlier, people dyed their hair ages before there was such a thing as a company called Clairol—or a salon exclusive enough to put you on a 2 month waiting list. How did they pull it off back then? By taking advantage of the natural dyes found in many plants and foods. Henna, to cite perhaps the prominent example, is a dye extracted from the ancient Oriental shrub of the same name. Women have used henna for centuries to dye both fingernails and hair. When applied as a hair dye, henna typically confers an auburn tint, which can be enhanced by the addition of ground teas, ground coffees, and conditioners. These additives are used to increase the brilliance of the ensuing color.

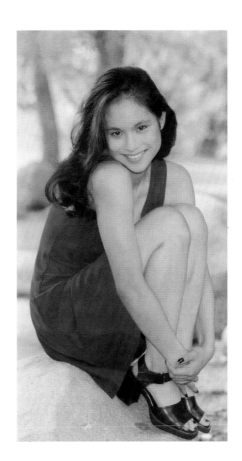

Don't be fooled, however, into thinking that henna is somehow milder or gentler than man-made dyes simply because it is "natural." Ma Nature can pack a powerful punch, and the fact is that most henna-based dyes qualify as fairly strong semipermanent dyes. They produce darker coloring than most novices initially suspect, and are notorious for producing stubborn stains on skin, nails, and clothes when not applied careful-ly. To use henna properly, choose a color that is somewhat lighter than the shade you're hoping to attain. Also, it's smart to protect your skin from inadvertent staining by smearing some Vaseline or Chap Stick on your earlobes, on the back of your neck, and along the hairline prior to applying the dye.

In addition to henna, many other natural substances possess qualities that are beneficial to the hair. A few of the more popu-lar (and proved!) of nature's hair care cures include:

- lemon juice, which can be applied (in diluted form) as a leave-in rinse to lighten dark blonde hair in the summer-time
- finely ground coffee or tea, which when mixed with warm water and conditioner stains the hair a rich brown color
- malt vinegar, or a cold rinse of either orange pekoe tea or tea containing rose hips, are known to enhance the color of red hair
- almond or soy oil, either of which can be mixed with a strong conditioner to improve the appearance of severely dry or damaged hair
- avocados, which can be mashed into a paste and applied to the hair as a conditioner

DANDRUFF

Dandruff is a generic term used to describe a variety of conditions that give rise to inflammation and scaling of the scalp—the familiar itching and flaking depicted so dramatically in shampoo commercials. Contrary to popular belief, the problem isn't caused by failure to wash the hair frequently enough, or by overly dry hair, or by dry scalp, or by using the wrong shampoo. The real culprit is a specific strain of yeast[7] called *Pityrosporum ovale*, which thrives amid the forest of hair follicles on our scalp and feeds on the bacteria-rich sebum that lubricates the hair roots. Now, the presence of this yeast on the scalp isn't restricted solely to dandruff sufferers; all of us play host to *Pityrosporum ovale* to one degree or another. But people with dandruff seem to be more sensitive to it.

When the yeast finds itself on a sensitive scalp, it sends the cell turnover rate into hyperdrive, which in turn produces the flaking that characterizes dandruff—and drives us nuts whenever we wear black or navy! The flakes themselves are actually particles of dead skin that have been prematurely shed from the uppermost layer of the scalp owing to the rapid generation of new cells. And, while everyone sports a new scalp every month or so, dandruff sufferers can rip through a full cellular replacement cycle in half the normal time.

Lumped into the same category as people with bad breath or body odor, folks with dandruff are often treated as if they had an infectious disease. The assumptions underlying this point of view, of course, are not only unfounded but unfair as well. Fortunately, our new understanding of how the condition originates and develops makes modern dandruff treatments far more effective than those that were available even just a few years ago. In the past, descaling agents and cortisone were used to address the scalp inflammation associated with various types of dandruff. Today's treatments, on the other hand, focus not only on controlling dandruff symptoms (inflammation, itchy scalp, flaking) but also on curbing the proliferation of the offending yeast, which is more at the root of the problem. These treatments range from over-the-counter shampoos containing traditional remedies such as sulfur, salicylic acid, antiseptic agents, or tar (yes, tar!), to stronger medicated shampoos and lotions that must be prescribed by your dermatologist. The drug *ketoconazole*, which has been used for decades to subdue many kinds of fungi, is now routinely recommended by dermatologists because of its efficacy in killing *Pityrosporum*. It can be found in prescribed products such as Nizoral™, a shampoo that contains the drug in a two percent concentration. Nizoral™ has proved so effective that it can, in many instances, stop dandruff-induced itching and flaking within just 2 weeks.

On the downside, even the best modern medications cannot banish the yeast entirely, so dandruff remains a chronic condition for which there is, as yet, no definitive cure. Like problem acne, this common disorder comes and goes at intervals, and must be dealt with as outbreaks occur. If you suffer from dandruff periodically, the single best move you can make is to see your dermatologist when a flare-up first arises so that he or she can determine the type and severity of dandruff that afflicts you, and then take appropriate steps to treat it.

Problem Dandruff: Seborrheic Dermatitis

While one person in two experiences occasional bouts of dandruff, some fifteen percent of Americans can blame their flaking on *seborrheic dermatitis* (or seborrhea, for short), a form of dandruff that often produces very severe itching and flaking. Seborrheic dermatitis is probably the most common rash known to humans. It can show up just about anyplace on the body, but appears most frequently in regions where the sebaceous glands are densely concentrated, such as the scalp, the T-zone, the eyebrows, and the chest. Like regular dandruff, seborrheic dermatitis can't be cured for keeps. It may go into remission for a while, but once you stop treatment it will probably come back. If untreated, this kind of severe dandruff can worsen to the point that the sufferer sheds not only flakes but hair as well. Yikes!

PRODUCT SPOTLIGHT   Dandruff Shampoos

Today's health-and-beauty consumer enjoys a broad selection of effective, over-the-counter shampoos that will not only clean the hair nicely but also help alleviate the worst symptoms of dandruff, seborrhea, and psoriasis[8] of the scalp. Our list of favorites includes Head & Shoulders by Procter & Gamble, DHS-Zinc by Person & Covey, Ionil Plus by Healthpoint, Neutrogena T-Gel, and Neutrogena T-Sal.

For best results, you will need to experiment a little. First, try several of the above products until you find three or four that lather up to your satisfaction and leave your hair feeling soft and shiny. Then, alternate brands from one washing to the next, and, most important, always allow the shampoo lather to stand on the scalp for at least 5 minutes before rinsing. After a week or two, your dandruff flakes should be gone. If not, you need to visit your dermatologist, who will probably recommend a prescription-strength shampoo like Nizoral or a prescribed topical medication.

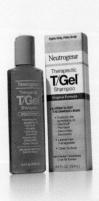
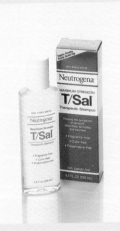

Left:
There are a wide variety of effective treatments for dandruff.

END NOTES

1. You'll recall from Chapter Five that scalp hair counts are linked closely to your natural hair color, and range from a low of 60,000 to 90,000 for the average redhead, to 100,000 to 130,000 for the typical blonde. Brown or black hair generally falls somewhere between these two extremes. In addition, straight hairs are usually thinner than curly or kinky hairs. The earlier discussion can be found in the section entitled "Blondes Have More . . . Hair!" on page 122.

2. Much in the manner that epidermal cells join together almost seamlessly to present a smooth, even surface in healthy, undamaged skin.

3. The word "additive" has developed something of a bad reputation these days, mainly because it is used most often in connection with food and so conjures up images of artificial flavorings, preservatives, and other things the health experts warn us against. But when it comes to shampoos, additives are usually included in the formula to achieve a specific cosmetic goal, such as plumping up the hair shafts or enhancing their lustre.

4. In this respect, as in many others, the principles of selecting the right shampoo are similar to those used in choosing the right skin cleanser.

5. Stabilizers are used in shampoos (and in other skin and hair care items) to create a nice consistency and to prevent the product from gumming up or hardening in the bottle.

6. The words *basic* and *caustic* are synonymous with alkaline in scientific terminology. So if you see these used to describe a hair care product, it means the product has a high pH.

7. Yeast results when minute cells of fungi clump together and form a frothy, semiliquid growth. Such growths can be readily found over the entire surface of our skin and along the linings of our mucous membranes. Skin irritation, inflammation, and/or infections occur when the pace of yeast growth outstrips the body's capacity to ward off the fungal invasion, or when an individual is especially sensitive to a certain strain of yeast.

8. A chronic (or recurring) skin disorder that results in localized patches of thick, inflamed, scale-encrusted skin. The disease, which can be distinguished from similar conditions like seborrhea by its trademark silver scales, most often strikes the scalp, elbows, and knees, though other areas on the torso are sometimes affected as well.

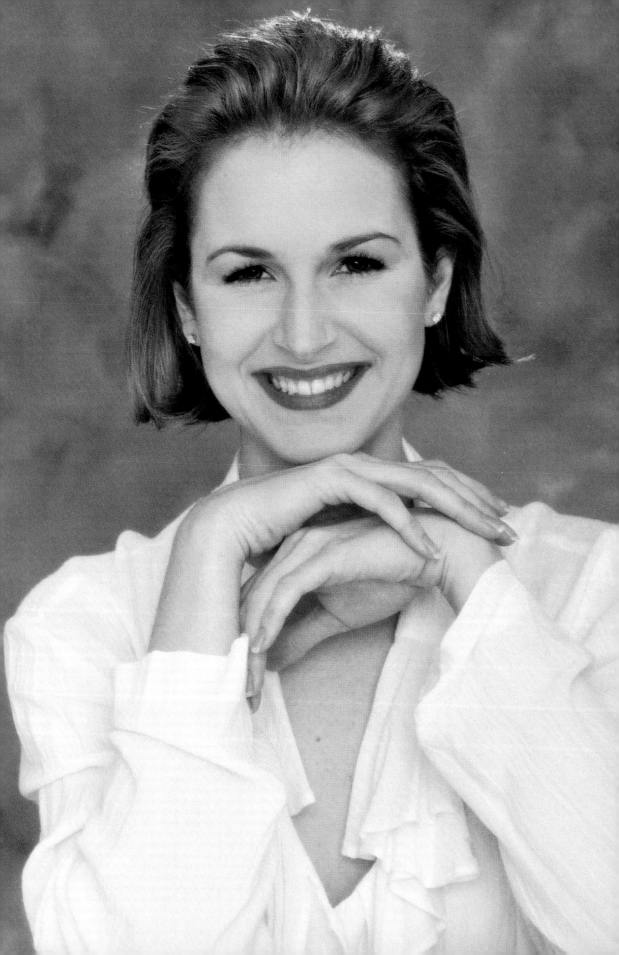

Nail It!
10 Perfect Fingers,
10 Perfect Toes

The elusive perfect 10: We all want it. We all know it's out there. But most of us never quite nail it. "It," of course, is the elegant, finished look of hands and feet that reach an aesthetically satisfying conclusion in the form of strong, shapely, well-groomed nails. No less than a glowing, unblemished complexion or firm, well-toned muscles, beautiful nails not only improve a woman's overall appearance but also testify to the world that their owner cares enough about herself to attend to every detail . . . right down to the tips of her fingers and toes. So have them we must. *But how?*

Too many of us, unfortunately, think that great looking nails can only be had by incredibly good genetic luck or by regular visits to an expensive salon. Not so! There are plenty of normal, everyday women with absolutely gorgeous nails who couldn't give you the name or phone number of a nail salon if their life depended on it. These women don't possess any secret wisdom or special training, either. They simply know how to care for and beautify their nails properly, using the very same implements and nail care products that are probably stowed away in your medicine cabinet or cosmetics bag right now. Read on—and find out how you, too, can achieve digital perfection!

NAIL FUNCTION

Below:

The way you care for your hands is a direct reflection of the way you care for yourself in general.

Nails, at first glance, look simple enough. If you didn't know better, you might assume they were similar to bones or cartilage, which, like nails, are relatively hard and tough. But as we discovered in Chapter One, nails are an extension of the skin. Like the softer skin that covers the face and body, the primary function of fingernails and toenails, at least biologically, is to provide protection to the tips of the fingers and toes—a purpose for which they are remarkably well suited. Additionally, nails refine your sense of touch, allow you to pick up small objects like paperclips and safety pins, and improve your ability to perform precise tasks such as threading a needle, sliding a dollar bill into a vending machine or scratching the winning number off your lottery ticket.

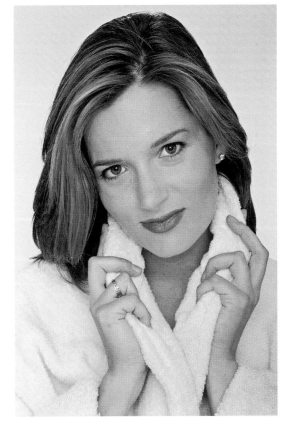

NAIL STRUCTURE

The tough outer portion of the nail—the part you trim, file, polish, and buff—is called the *nail plate*. You might be surprised to learn that the nail plate is composed chiefly of keratin, the same structural protein found not only in hair but also in the epidermal layer of "regular" skin. The keratin in your nails, however, contains more sulfur[1] than the keratin in your hair and skin; and it is this high sulfur content that gives the nails their hardness. Now, keratin—whether of the hard variety found in your nails or the soft variety found in your skin's epidermis—is a protein that likes to layer. Consequently, the nail plate, like the epidermis, is a layered affair, a fact you can observe for yourself if you look very closely at the cut portion of a clipped toenail. Fatty acids called *phospholipids* in the upper and lower layers of the nail plate provide the resilience and flexibility that enable the nail to bend some without breaking.

The nail plate itself, by the way, is not alive, and thus cannot be "fed," "nourished," or "replenished" with anything you'll encounter on a drugstore or supermarket shelf. Like the hair shaft, it is an inorganic (or non-living) outgrowth produced by a nucleus of living, reproductive cells at its base. This collection of live cells is known as the *nail matrix*. Most of the nail matrix lies hidden from view beneath the *posterior nail fold* at the back of each nail. But a small, white, crescent-shaped segment of it called the *lunula* can be seen near the nail base.

Two other important parts of the nail are the *cuticle* and the *nail bed*. The cuticle, as you probably know, is an opaque (or semitransparent) skin fold at the base of the nail plate. This tender, delicate, slightly scrunched lip of dead skin performs a pair of vital functions: First, it connects and secures the nail plate to the skin of the finger or toe to which it belongs; and second, it shields the vulnerable nail base from foreign objects and infection. If you're one of those women who find cuticles unattractive, you'll want to exercise real care and caution when you try to push them out of sight. Your nails need the protection offered by the cuticles, and they are easily damaged by trimming (a definite don't) and overly aggressive pushing and prodding (which, if it must be done at all, should be done gently, as we'll demonstrate shortly).

The nail bed, for its part, is a soft, thick layer of grooved tissue that lies beneath the nail plate and acts as a sort of "shock absorber" for the nail above. When someone, say, steps on your big toe at a dance or accidentally closes a door on the tips of your fingers, the resulting damage to the nail is minimized—

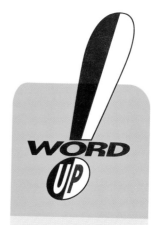

WORD UP

Lunula is a Latin word that means "half-moon," an apt description of the only visible portion of the nail matrix.

though by no means eliminated—by the cushioning effect of the bed. In addition, the nail bed shelters the extensive network of tiny blood vessels that carry necessary nutrients and oxygen to the nail matrix, as well as the sensitive nerve endings that let your brain know what's new and exciting at the outermost extremities of the body.

NAIL GROWTH: BY THE NUMBERS

The nail matrix, unlike its counterpart in the hair, never gets a chance to "rest," because nails don't grow in cycles; they grow constantly. Fingernails grow at a clip (if you'll pardon the pun!) of ⅛ to ¼ inch per month; toenails, about two to three times more slowly. Though growth rates vary from one individual to the next, it takes the average Joe or Jane around 6 months to grow a full fingernail, and 12 to 18 months to grow a full toenail, as anyone unlucky enough to have lost one of either could tell you. The rate of nail growth tapers off as we age, but almost never, ever shuts down entirely,[2] even when the nail matrix suffers severe damage. Thus, when the health of the matrix becomes compromised—whether through direct injury, infection, or extreme malnutrition—the typical result is slowed or

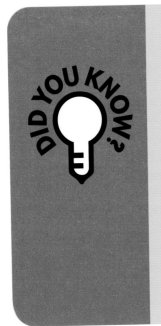

Fingernails—like retirees—seem to favor warm weather. Nail growth rates, for reasons unknown to researchers, typically heat up in the summer and cool down in the winter. But don't pack away those clippers just because it's snowing outside: Changes in seasonal growth rates aren't *that* dramatic!

Some other interesting morsels: In most people, the nails of the right hand grow faster than the nails of the left, and growth rates vary from finger to finger. The general rule of thumb (ouch! . . . sorry, couldn't resist!) is that the longer the finger is, the faster its nail grows. Thus the nail of the middle finger grows fastest; the ring finger, next fastest; the index finger next. Nail growth rates also accelerate during pregnancy and immediately after an illness.

deformed nail growth rather than no growth at all. Funky look-ing, misshapen nails or nails that grow in odd directions usual-ly indicate that the matrix is not functioning as it should.

Memo to Office Staff . . .

Don't be shocked if the secretaries and data entry specialists at your place of work own some of the strongest, healthiest nails in the building. You see, it seems as though there's something about the repetitive clicking of a keyboard that just drives the nail matrix crazy, stimulating it to produce new growth quicker than it does under ordinary circumstances. Likewise, the nails of most pianists grow at a faster than normal pace, even though you'd think the incessant pounding of the keys would instead cause splitting and breakage.

Nail Growth & Your Diet

While your nails may reward time spent at the keyboard by growing faster, they don't appear to care much one way or the other about what you eat or the dietary supplements you take. You may have heard, for instance, that loading up on gelatin capsules, calcium pills, or certain vitamins will lead to longer, stronger nails. Or that a nice, hearty serving of seaweed or spinach will give your nails the iron they "need." But these are myths, pure and simple—just like the myths that attempt to link specific foods with outbreaks of acne. Your nails, remem-ber, are no more alive than the hairs on your head, so the foods and supplements you ingest cannot positively affect them in any measurable way.

Sadly enough, the only known effect your diet can have on the nails is to make them weak or deformed, as sometimes hap-pens in cases of severe malnutrition, crash dieting, or binge-purge eating. But aside from these exceptional situations, it's almost a certainty that your present diet provides adequate amounts of the vitamins and minerals required by the nails to reach their natural potential in terms of both growth and strength. Thus, if we consider only the health of the nails—and ignore the rest of the body[3]—what you eat can hurt, but cannot help, your nails.

NAIL BREAKERS

Despite its hard, glossy surface, the nail plate does not form a completely impenetrable barrier to the outside world. It is, in reality, a porous structure, capable of absorbing external substances such as water, nail polish pigment, and chemicals from nail cosmetics and household cleansers, to cite just a few examples. Once these substances find their way below the outer surface of the nail plate, the affected nail can become dry, stressed, and prone to breakage. In some instances, complete nail loss can result, especially when a very adverse reaction occurs or when powerful chemicals penetrate into sensitive areas like the nail folds or cuticle.

Overwashing Your Hands

Water ranks as the substance absorbed in the greatest quantity by the nails, and for the majority of people causes few really big problems. But when exposure to moisture becomes too frequent—as it can for people who, for example, wash their hands several times a day or swim daily—the nails inevitably suffer. They take on water and expand when wet, then lose moisture and shrink as they dry. Constant repetition of this cycle of expansion and contraction eventually weakens the nails, rendering them very susceptible to breakage.

Who is at risk for this type of nail damage? Basically, anyone who overwashes their hands, whether of necessity or because of a compulsion to be ultra-clean. In the necessity category, we may include everyone whose job requires frequent hand washing, such as food service and restaurant workers, waitresses, bartenders, nurses, dental assistants, hair stylists, and so on. To minimize shrinkage and stress, always rinse your hands thoroughly after washing to remove residual soap, and when possible treat your nails with petroleum jelly or a rich, moisturizing hand lotion while they are still slightly damp. This will help seal in the moisture needed for healthy nails, plus prevent your hands from becoming dry and chapped. Some products to try: Neutrogena New Hands, BeautiControl Skinlogics Hand and Nail Therapy, and Develop 10 Nourishment for Nails and Skin.

Working Your Nails to the Nubs
With Common Household Cleansers

Household cleansers and disinfectants also chip away at nail health, and are notorious for causing dryness and brittleness. The simple fix here is to wear rubber or latex gloves while you're wiping, shining, scouring, or scrubbing. Gloves, in fact, are a great idea for several different reasons: First, they insulate the nails and hands from harsh and potentially irritating chemical agents; second, they protect against the accidental nail breakage and chipping of polish that occur so often during vigorous manual work; and third, they shield your skin and nails from the legions of microbes that inhabit countertops, cooking

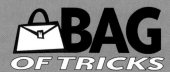

How To Stay Stain-Free With Dark Polish

While the very idea of yellow nails may be enough to make you gag, there is absolutely no good reason to limit yourself exclusively to the paler side of the nail polish spectrum. If your favorite dark polish discolors, try one or both of these simple solutions:

1. Switch brands or shades. Some specific brands and shades tend to seep pigment more readily than others, so you may well be able to solve your problem by merely trying a new brand or using one shade lighter (or even darker) in color with the same brand.

2. Use whatever brand or shade you like, but always put down a clear base coat (or better yet, two) before applying dark pol-

ish. This is the dull, foolproof, works-every-time kind of fix preferred by those who, like us, don't want to wonder what we'll uncover once the polish has been removed. Hey, salons use base coats. Why shouldn't you?

A word of caution, though: If a nail turns yellow, you shouldn't automatically assume that dark polish is the culprit. Some very nasty yeast infections also promote yellowing. If the yellowed nail begins to separate from its bed or becomes thick and crusty, you're probably dealing with an infection and need to see your dermatologist right away for treatment.

surfaces, sinks, toilets, and other germ-friendly areas around the house. For optimal nail health, you should really wear gloves not only when you clean house, but whenever you handle strong chemicals (as when you strip or stain a piece of furniture) or do rough work of any kind (such as gardening or waxing the car).

The Darker Side of Some Nail Polish Shades

Nail cosmetics comprise yet another category in the list of potential nail wreckers. Polishes, surprisingly enough, are far from being the worst offenders, despite the staggering number of different brands, shades, and styles currently produced. Fact is, most polishes coexist quite happily with the nails, with the exception of certain deep shades of brown, red, black and purple, which occasionally discolor the nails after removal. The discoloration takes place when pigment from the polish seeps into the nail plate[4] and leaves behind a yellowish cast even after the entire surface coat has been removed. This yellowing, though admittedly unattractive, generally amounts to nothing more than a temporary nuisance, and the nails gradually regain their natural color as new growth replaces old. In the meantime, you can lighten the discoloration by buffing stained nails with a stiff-bristled brush and then washing with warm, soapy water.[5]

The "Brittle" Truth About Nail Polish Removers

While the great majority of polishes are relatively harmless to the nails, the same cannot be said for many polish removers. These products, no matter how cleverly formulated or well manufactured, are essentially modified paint strippers, as even the faintest whiff of an open bottle attests. Is it any wonder, then, that they can be drying and irritating to the nails and surrounding skin? In fact, if polish removers were any gentler, they probably wouldn't work as effectively—or smell as badly—as they do!

Acetone & Nail Damage

Acetone, a solvent used in many popular brands of polish remover, is often singled out as a prime suspect when a woman's nails show evidence of excessive dryness and brittleness. The reputation is at least partly deserved, since acetone is known to cause adverse reactions in some people and to weaken nails from the inside out if overused. In fairness, however, it's worth noting that any solvent strong enough to chemically dissolve nail polish is, by its very nature, likely to be drying and potentially damaging to the nails, *regardless of what the label may say to the contrary*. Nail polishes and enamels, like the paint on your house or the stain on your Mom's antique dresser, are made to be tough and long-lasting. So it takes serious stuff to make them vanish with a few swipes of a cotton ball soaked in remover. What's more, even products labeled as acetone-free are not always safe for people sensitive to it, because acetone derivatives such as acetate are commonly used as replacements and thus produce results similar to those of the better known ingredient.

Give Your Nails a Break . . .

by exercising a little moderation and leaving them uncovered every so often. Overuse of polish remover, in particular—and of nail care products, in general—is far and away the leading cause of cracked, damaged nails.

DAMAGE CONTROL FOR DRIED-OUT NAILS

If you've learned through "brittle" experience that your nails and skin are sensitive to acetone, of course it makes good sense to look for a polish remover that contains neither acetone nor solvents derived from it. But let's say your polish remover is genuinely acetone-free, yet your nails are still as brittle and breakable as overfried bacon. What then? The first—and most drastic—solution is to quit wearing polish altogether. Sure, this isn't a great option. But if your nails can't tolerate remover without falling to pieces, why even bother to polish them in the first place?

A second remedy—and one that cures many nail ills—is to limit your use of both polish and remover. For starters, never apply polish remover more than once a week, and give your nails a brief 2- or 3-day vacation from all polishes and nail cosmetics at least a couple of times a month. If that doesn't work, try the same program with an acetone-free remover that's loaded

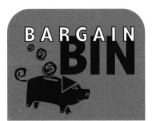

BARGAIN BIN

Olive oil is a low-cost, hypoallergenic way to moisturize and soften dry, brittle nails. Try it as an alternative to more expensive moisturizing creams and lotions.

with moisturizing agents to counteract the drying effects of the product's solvent.

Finally, many women overcome dryness and brittleness by soaking their fingertips in warm water or olive oil (yes, the same stuff you mix with vinegar for Italian salad dressing!) for 10 minutes every evening. If you soak in warm water, lightly pat the nails dry—but not completely dry—with a washcloth or towel, then apply a thick moisturizing cream or lotion to your still-damp nails. If you soak in olive oil, the oil itself is your moisturizer. Simply work it into the nails with gentle rubbing when you're through soaking, and dab off any excess with a tissue or cotton ball.

GOING WITH THE PROS: SALON MANICURES & PEDICURES

Most women regard a professional manicure or pedicure as a special treat, so even if you can't afford to visit a salon weekly or monthly, don't be afraid to schedule an appointment occasionally. Trust us, the salon will be happy for the business, and even irregular visits can be both fun and instructive for you. Often a good nail technician will not only make your nails attractive for the present, but also teach you the essentials of maintaining the look between appointments.

Salons, however, are not especially well regulated for sanitation and hygiene. Sure, government standards have been established, but day-to-day enforcement of them is lax in most places, and next to nonexistent in others. As a result, you can't assume that a particular business is clean and safe just because it's listed under "Salons" in the phone book. And, while a good nail salon poses virtually no health risks for its clients, an unclean one can expose you to everything from mild bacterial and fungal infections of the nails, to extremely dangerous diseases such as hepatitis and HIV.

What To Look For in a Nail Salon

Since you have to be your own watchdog, it's important to recognize how a salon with sound sanitary practices is run. When you visit, here's what you should see:

- Clean towels and a container of EPA (Environmental Protection Agency)-registered, hospital-grade disinfectant (for storing metal tools) on every nail technician's table. Very few states require complete submersion of metal implements, but the better salons will do so anyhow.

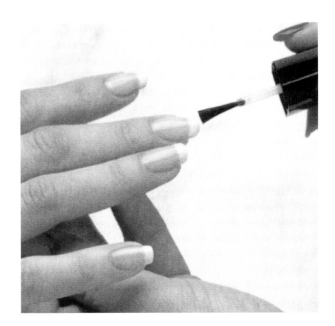

- Thorough washing and disinfection of all tools after *every* use. Make sure the washing is done with hot, soapy water (not just a rinse), and that disinfectant is applied not only to the working portions of implements but to the handles as well. In addition, emery boards should be discarded after every use to prevent transmission of yeast or bacterial infections from one client's nails to the next.
- Cleaning and disinfection of work tables and other nearby surfaces after every manicure or pedicure.
- Washing of hands by both the technician and the client just prior to treatment. Hands should be washed with sanitizing foam, not ordinary bar soap.
- A smoke-free environment. Many nail-care products are highly flammable, so smoking–even by clients—should not be permitted. An overwhelming smell of nail polish or polish remover, incidentally, signals inadequate ventilation and an increased fire hazard.

THE ULTIMATE AT-HOME MANICURE: NAIL IT IN SIX EASY STEPS!

Salon care, for all its diehard advocates, requires an outlay of money and time that many folks would just as soon devote to other purposes. In fact, the majority of women fall into this camp. They do their own manicures and pedicures at home, in some instances with results that rival those produced by the very best nail technicians. And you can, too, with just a little guidance, a few basic implements, and of course a lot of practice. Who knows? You might become so skilled that you'd never trust your fingers and toes to anyone else again!

Getting Started & Gearing Up

To do your nails like a pro, you need to act like a pro. That means owning the right gear and working in an environment that is as clean and antiseptic as you can make it. Let's begin with a list of necessary items:

- Isopropyl rubbing alcohol: to be used for disinfecting implements; look for 70 percent or higher alcohol content.
- Cotton balls or roll of uncut cotton. Prepackaged cotton balls are the more convenient choice, but the roll is cheaper in the long run, and allows you to cut pieces to the exact size and shape you need.
- Orange stick.
- Emery board or diamond file.
- Toenail clippers.
- Pair of small, sharp manicure scissors: for trimming hangnails.
- Base coat: to help polish adhere and to fill in cracks, pits, ridges, and other surface irregularities.
- Nail hardener or strengthener (optional): use only if your nails have a tendency to split, crack or peel. A few of the older-style hardeners and strengtheners still contain the preservative formaldehyde, a chemical known to cause allergic reactions with alarming frequency. Be sure that yours doesn't.
- Polish in several colors: a few basics such as clear, coral pink, and rose red are musts, but beyond that you are limited only by your imagination, your budget, and the restrictions imposed by your natural skin and hair coloring. To prevent washed-out color during those bare-toed summer months, choose formulations with built-in sunscreen, which makes the polish stable in UV light.
- Sealing coat: also called a top coat. Used to add glossiness to—and improve the durability of—the enamel or colored nail polish you apply.

Your Work Area: Sanitation & Safety

Cleanliness and sanitation are no less important in your home than in a salon, perhaps even more so, seeing as how you live there. Yet, while most of us live in neat, tidy quarters, the environment may not be antiseptic (or germ-free) as it ought to be for a full manicure or pedicure. Here are a few pointers to get you headed in the right direction.

- If you'll be working in the bathroom, try to perform your manicure or pedicure immediately after the room has been thoroughly cleaned and disinfected. The germs that thrive in dirty toilet bowls and messy sinks, after all, aren't necessarily the kind you want to invite to your cuticles for a dinner party.

- Clean and sterilize all of your tools just as if you were employed at a professional salon (see above for details). Ideally, tools should be cleaned before *and* after each treatment. Isopropyl rubbing alcohol can serve as your alternative to the hospital-grade disinfectant used at salons.

- Don't use the same emery board over and over again. An old board can pick up germs just lying around in your purse, medicine cabinet, or cosmetics bag; and a dull board, like a dull razor, is actually more likely to damage your nails than a sharp one.

- Keep your hands away from your eyes, ears, lips, and nose during the course of the manicure or pedicure. Most allergic reactions to nail polish, for example, don't result from the effect of dried polish on the nails, but from wet polish that has accidentally come in contact with the sensitive skin around the eyes. And as for polish remover, we'll just quote a common warning found on the back of many bottles: **Harmful to synthetic fabrics, wood finishes, and plastics.** If the stuff can do damage to wood and plastic, just imagine how even a smidgeon of it would feel in the corner of an eye. Yeowww!

- If you must smoke during the course of your manicure, do so OUTSIDE while your nails are drying, far removed from potentially flammable substances like polish remover. Or better yet, don't smoke at all!

Now that you're ready to start, the first question on your mind might well be: How often should I do my nails? Our reply: Probably more often than you think. Unless your nails grow very slowly, a weekly manicure is a beauty must. For pedicures, you can space treatments every 2 to 3 weeks, owing to the slower growth rate of toenails versus fingernails. Let your nails go longer than these guidelines and our feeling is that they will have grown out to the extent that no amount of touching up will look good. Of course, they're your nails, your hands, your feet. Check 'em out after the suggested amount of time has passed, then decide if you're comfortable with the look or not. The one redeeming virtue of the at-home manicure or pedicure—beyond the satisfaction of having done it yourself—is that takes just 15 or 20 minutes to do both hands (or feet) once you've become adept at it—a small price to pay when weighed against the $15 to $35 you would have paid for the same treatment at a good salon.

Step 1: Removing Old Polish

Remove existing polish with a moisturizing polish remover like Sally Hansen Pro Vitamin B_5 Acetone-Free Nail Polish Remover. To soften the old polish, apply a cotton ball or cotton pad lightly saturated with polish remover to the nail and hold it there for a few seconds. Then, wipe from the base of the nail outward until every trace of polish is gone. After you've done all ten nail plates, clean up any remnants of old polish that are still clinging to the cuticles and nail folds with a cotton ball lightly moistened (but not saturated) with polish remover. Since these are sensitive areas, you want to use as little polish remover on them as possible.

Step 2: Filing

Reshape the nails with an emery board, using the fine side of the board. *Do not* file back and forth in a sawing motion. Instead, always file in one direction, exerting gentle, even pressure. Angle the board against the bottom edge of the nail, and work from one side (far left or far right) to the other. This helps prevent splitting.

When all ten nails have been filed to your satisfaction, soak your fingertips in warm water for 10 minutes or so. This will not only rehydrate your nails and thus counteract the drying effects of polish remover, but also soften your cuticles in preparation for Step 3.

A Few Tips To File Away...

Overall, filing beats clipping hands down as a method for trimming and shaping the fingernails, because it's less stressful to the nail plate. Improper filing, however, can lead to both nail trauma and displeasing aesthetic results. Translation: You could crack or break your nails, and they could wind up looking positively horrid!

To file correctly, hold your emery board at a 45-degree to the nail's edge and, as we've noted, work in a single direction from one edge to the other. Square-tipped nails are stronger than tapered ones, so file straight across the tips if your nails are at all prone to peeling or splitting. For the same reason, be careful not to over-round the nails near the edges, and never file downward at the sides. Lastly, don't get near your nails with a file unless they've grown out enough to maintain a good, solid base at the bottom.

Step 3: Cuticle Care

Our best medical advice is that you leave your cuticles alone. But since so few people actually follow this guidance, we feel obligated to tell how to care for them as gently and safely as possible. Here's how: Soften the cuticles with warm-water soaking, a rich moisturizer, or cuticle oil, according to your preference. Once the cuticles have been softened, gently push them from view with the tip of a finger (not the edge of a nail!) or an orange stick. If you have any hangnails, clip them at this point with a small pair of manicure scissors, following the guidelines below. Next, buff your nails thoroughly, and clean under the nail tips with an orange stick wrapped in wet cotton.

Below:
Keeping your hands well-moisturized helps prevent dry, ragged cuticles.

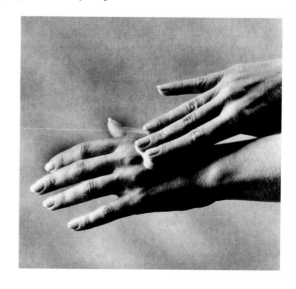

Hangnails

A hangnail is a small strip of skin that has become separated from the nail fold or cuticle. Hangnails can be surprisingly painful, and are typically caused by nail biting, nail chewing, accidental ripping of the skin, or incorrect use of nail implements such as orange sticks or cuticle pushers. To treat a hangnail, snip away the detached skin flap with manicure scissors, and promptly apply a topical antibiotic such as polysporin and bacitracin to prevent infection. When you snip, *be extremely careful to avoid cutting the cuticle or nail fold*, as doing so will not only cause the cuticle to grow back thicker and coarser, but also greatly increase your risk of infection.

If you accidentally cut yourself while treating a hangnail or manipulating your cuticles, keep a very close eye on the injury. If it shows any sign of infection or doesn't heal fully and cleanly within a day or two, see your dermatologist for help.

Step 4: Applying Base Coat

Place one hand—palm down, fingers outspread—flat on the table. With the other hand, apply the base coat of your choosing. A well-applied base will not only make your polish stick better, but also allow it to coat more evenly and smoothly by filling in any surface irregularities. Two thin layers of base coat, incidentally, work better than one heavier layer. If you experience problems with splitting, cracking, or peeling of the nails, you may also want to apply a nail hardener or strengthener as your second coat. Your strengthener can be used to coat the entire nail, or applied solely to the nail tips, where these problems typically occur. Tru Nails Professional and Sally Hansen both sell very effective, salon-quality strengtheners that can be found at better beauty supply stores.

Brushing Up on the Basics of Applying Base & Color

- Allow one coat to dry completely before you apply the next one.
- Always brush from the base of the nail to the tip, using just enough polish to cover without build-up, and working from the center of the nail to the sides.
- Cover the entire nail with a thin, even coat.

- Avoid brushing base or color into the nail folds and cuticles as much as possible.
- To prevent chipping, remove just a hairline of polish from the edge of the treated nail by running your opposite thumb along it.
- A warm shower or foot soaking is the easiest, safest way to clean up polish that has strayed outside the fingernails or toenails. The moisture and heat will peel the excess polish right off.

Step 5: Applying Color

If you choose to color your nails, apply two coats of polish to achieve deep, full, chip-resistant color. Again, as with your base, you'll be better served if you don't just glob the stuff on. Thickly coated color likes to chip and crack. Think thin—and think even! Work from the base of the nail to the tip, center to sides, and be careful to avoid brushing polish into the nail folds or cuticle. This can make your nails look ragged around the edges, and can be a real pain to repair unless you start over from square one. Plus, it's always best to keep both polish and remover away from these easily irritated areas.

So Many Coats, So Little Time...

If you apply base, color, and sealing coats according to our guidelines, you'll wind up with four to five sheer layers of polish on your nails, each of which takes several minutes to dry thoroughly. Though it may be tempting to save yourself some time by applying just two coats (say, one each of base and color), we can assure you that the resulting manicure will not be as attractive or as durable as it could be. More layers, as long as they are properly applied, mean stronger nails, a longer-lasting manicure, and better retention of necessary moisture, which is why almost all nail salons favor a multilayer treatment.

Since it doesn't pay to cut down on the number of coats you apply, the key is to minimize the time you spend waiting for each separate coat to dry. There are two very painless ways to go about this: One, soak your just-brushed nails in ice water to help the recently applied polish set more quickly. While you won't be able to use your hands as if the polish were completely air dried, your nails will be ready to accept the next coat in fairly short order. Second, choose one of the many quick-setting, quick-drying polishes now on the market.

Choosing Your Nail Color

One of the more enjoyable aspects of applying color is, of course, selecting the shade you want to wear. We won't pretend to tell you what color your nails should be under all circumstances. So much, in the end, depends on your skin and hair coloring, the other makeup you're wearing, your clothes, the season, the occasion, and the overall effect you're trying to achieve. But we will say this much: Allow yourself to have some fun! You could wear a different color every day of the coming year, and not scratch the surface of what's available these days. Metallics, glitters, offbeat pastels, and hues too weird for words now share the stage with the corals and clears and roses and rubies that used to dominate department store displays. So, even though it's wise to have a few basic shades that will take you anywhere, anytime (as we advise below), don't let yourself get stuck in a one-color rut. Experiment. Be creative. Take a dare. You'll have a blast in the process, and possibly discover that colors you hardly considered before are actually just your style. You never can tell: The polish you try on a whim today could be the inspiration for the blouse or scarf you'll be wearing tomorrow!

If you're in the mood to stir things up colorwise, check out Mini Pots of Color by Creative Nails. They're fun, funky, and *fairly* reasonably priced for a six-pot pack of multihued mischief.

The downside of using nail color creatively is that mistakes can and will be made every now and again. The most common: nail polish that clashes with either your lipstick or your clothes. For those times when you can't afford a mishap or simply don't wish to think too hard about what color to use, we recommend choosing two or three shades that blend well with the bulk of your wardrobe, or sticking to a pale pink that you can wear with everything but orange tones. Among the pinks, Revlon Ballet Buff, Essie Ballet Slippers and OPI Coney Island (an especially clear, non-Tinkerbell shade) are all as classical as Mozart, while

YSL #98, a pale opalescent lavender, takes racy right to the edge (but within the bounds) of good taste. For darker complected women, Cover Girl NailSlicks In The Buff and Elizabeth Arden Choco are two unassuming, yet flattering, shades that rarely disappoint.

Step 6: The Sealing Coat

Application of a sealing coat is the final step in your at-home manicure. Once your color (or clear) coat has dried, brush on sealer from the base of the nail to the tip. Carry the sealer all the way to the tip's edge and then over, so that a little coats the underside of the nail as well. A well-formulated sealer will not only protect the finish of your color coat but also enhance its glossiness.

The French Manicure

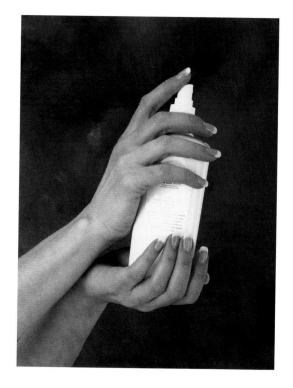

Above:
A French manicure.

It's 4 PM on Saturday afternoon. You're going out to a nice restaurant for dinner at 8 PM, so you'd like to do your nails, but haven't yet decided which dress you'll wear. Do you put off your nails until later? Or choose the dress now to be sure that your nail color complements it? Well, you can do either . . . *or neither!* A French manicure offers a clean, classic look that will go with any dress in your closet and absolutely never, ever seem out of place or give the appearance of an afterthought. The French style differs from an ordinary manicure in three simple, but significant respects:

1. The tips of the nails are filed square across, not rounded or tapered.
2. White polish is used to color the end of the tips. Depending on the length of your nails and your personal preference, the line of white on the tips may be so thin as to be barely noticeable, or may be as wide as $\frac{1}{8}$ to $\frac{1}{4}$ inch thick. Some women with exceptionally long nails (something we don't recommend) may go even wider. If you

opt for a wide strip of white, make sure you brush a smooth, straight line with a clean, sharp edge at the bottom. The white polish goes on over your base, but under the top coat.

3. Clear or very transparent pink polish is used to cover the entire nail, including the white tip. When your top coat has fully dried, buff to a natural shine. If you've done your work well, people will have to look very closely to know if you've applied polish—or simply possess the most naturally healthy, lustrous nails they've ever seen.

The Cut-Off Point for Nail Length

How long should you let your nails get? In general, no longer than ½ inch beyond the ends of your fingers. Long, spiky nails are impractical for day-to-day living, break easily, and almost always look disproportionate to the fingers and hand. If you are active in sports, do much housework, use a computer, or play the piano, you will be best to stop well shy of the ½ inch mark, and grow your nails out no more than ⅛ inch past the fingertips. This will give you enough nail to shape and color in an attractive, feminine manner, but not so much that you're constantly fumbling with everyday tasks merely to avoid incidental breakage.

ARTIFICIAL NAILS: A DECEPTIVELY PAINLESS SOLUTION

Many women who want longer or more finished-looking nails choose to use artificial nails—either because they feel their own nails are too soft or too brittle to sustain solid growth past the fingertip or because they wish to sidestep the constant care required to maintain a manicured look. Without a doubt, the promise of beautiful, maintenance-free nails is alluring, especially when every drugstore and discount department store in America carries press-on and glue-on nails that can be applied in a fraction of the time it takes to manicure the fingers of just one hand. But like so many other promises that sound too good to be true—think fad diets or "instant" ab machines—the easy route to the perfect 10 doesn't pan out as a healthy long-term solution.

Your natural nails, as you'll remember, are designed to be

porous. Furthermore, they are made to be exposed to the elements. When you cover them up and seal them in beneath a plastic or acrylic shell, moisture that would have otherwise evaporated harmlessly cannot escape. In a relatively short period of time, the nail plates can become saturated, soft, and loosely secured to their nail beds. You can even lose an entire nail this way, particularly if an infection develops while the nail plate loosens and softens. Additionally, the glues and adhesives used in artificial nails sometimes prove irritating to the nails and the surrounding skin of the nail folds and cuticles.

On the whole, we believe that artificial nails are a poor choice for most women, most of the time. You can, however, make an exception every now and again, as long as you confine yourself to using press-on nails—which seem to cause relatively few serious problems for their users—and strictly limit the number of days you wear them. How long is too long? Anything beyond 3 days, in our estimation. But don't fret. That's more than enough time to get you through a friend's wedding or homecoming weekend when your natural nails aren't looking their best.

Types of Artificial Nails

Several types of artificial nails are currently offered, both in salons and in stores. These differ widely in terms of cost, permanence, appearance, and method of application, but all share one trait in common: They can ultimately weaken and damage your natural nails, especially if you use them too often or leave them on for extended stretches.

- **Press-on nails** are made from pieces of preformed plastic, and utilize either an adhesive backing or a brush-on glue to attach the product to the nail plate. Press-ons have established a fairly good track record for safety: Compared to other types of artificial nails, they rarely cause allergic reactions or give rise to infections. The most common complaints about press-ons are that they tend to lose their grip after a few days of use, and they don't look as realistic or natural as, say, sculptured nails or nail wraps. They also sometimes pop off unexpectedly. Yet despite these shortcomings, a set of good quality press-on nails should serve quite nicely for the kind of limited, short-term usage we favor. They're inexpensive, easy-to-use, and available at nearly every store that carries cosmetics or health and beauty care products. Just be certain to select a color that doesn't look unnaturally glossy, and do some careful trimming of the plastic if any of the artificial nails are the slightest bit too large for your nail plates. This will not only help them adhere better, but also make them less likely to chafe and irritate your nail folds and cuticles.

- **Nail tips**, also known as glue-on nails, are made from acetate, and can be applied at a salon or at home. While you'll pay more for glue-on nails at a salon, the results will probably be better than if you use one of the at-home kits, since applying them properly can be difficult. Either way, though, a three-step process is employed: First, the acetate tip is trimmed to match the shape of the natural nail tip to which it will be affixed; second, the trimmed nail is attached with a special acrylate adhesive; and third, a mixture of acrylic powder and glue is layered on from the base of the nail to the bottom edge of the artificial tip so that the finished nail presents a smooth, even surface. Unlike press-on nails, glue-ons typically last (and look good) for several weeks if touched up with polish periodically. Some may consider this a benefit, but we actually view it as a drawback because the longer your natural nails are covered, the greater your risk of experiencing an adverse reaction or contracting a fungal infection. Air pockets often form between the nail plate and the artificial nail, and this creates a prime breeding ground for fungi. In addition, the strong adhesives used for nail tip treatments are known to prompt severe reactions in many women, including thickening of the nails, cracking, discoloration, and in the very worst cases, irreversible nail deformities.

- **Nail wraps** are strips of paper, silk, or linen that are custom trimmed to the size and shape of the full nail plate with just enough extra material at the free edge of the nail to slightly overlap the tip. Once the strips have been cut to size, they are carefully glued on and manicured with base coat, polish, and a top coat. The excess material at the tip is neatly tucked under the nail tip and glued as well. Nail wraps typically last 2 to 3 weeks, or about the time it takes your natural nails to slice through the wrapped edges. Like nail tips, wraps are difficult to apply at home (you're essentially one-handed!) and keep the nails covered too long to suit our taste.

- **Sculptured (or custom-molded) nails** are fashioned by placing a mold over the fingertips to outline the shape of your real nails, then brushing on layers of acrylic polymers[6] until the desired thickness and length are attained. The process, when done correctly by an experienced nail technician, results in an extremely realistic, long-lasting look that the salons like to advertise as a "permanent" cosmetic fix. What the salons won't tell you, however, is that the very permanence of the procedure only magnifies the potential problems associated with artificial nails in general, which include saturation and softness of the underlying nail plate, irritation to surrounding skin, allergic reactions, and susceptibility to infection. Facial eczema, intense pain in the fingertips, and lost nails are just a few of the nastier and all-too-common drawbacks to this expensive and ultimately crippling treatment. So while you may love your "new" nails today, odds are that your old nails will suffer serious and perhaps irreversible damage over the long haul.

YOUR AT-HOME PEDICURE

The steps we've described for your at-home manicure cover, in nearly every important respect, the essentials of performing a do-it-yourself pedicure. The lone exception is that toenails, owing to their thickness, should be clipped rather than filed when they exceed an acceptable length. Proper clipping of the toenails is a must not only for practical and aesthetic reasons, but also because it helps prevent the occurrence of ingrown nails, a common but painful condition that, if left unchecked, can require surgical treatment.

Ingrown Nails

An ingrown toenail occurs when the pointed corner of a nail becomes lodged in the sensitive skin of the nail fold, causing the affected area to become red, inflamed, and extremely tender. Most ingrown toenails develop due to improper cutting of the nail, though many also occur as a result of wearing shoes or socks that fit too tightly. To prevent ingrown toenails, you should...

- Purchase shoes and socks roomy enough to allow all five little piggies to move about freely without squealing in pain. Women's dress pumps, pointy-toed boots, and thick, tightly knit hosiery are all common piggy pinchers, so select carefully and take your time at the shoe store. Always try on both the left and right shoes in the pair (most of us have one foot that's slightly larger than the other), and walk around for a few minutes before making your decision. And even then, don't be reluctant to return shoes if you find that your toes feel cramped or bunched after the first full day or two you wear them. It's difficult to simulate real-life usage by merely pacing back and forth on a carpeted sales floor, and if the toe box is too narrow, no amount of "breaking in" or shoe stretching is likely to widen it adequately without damaging not only the shoes but your toes as well.

- Cut your toenails correctly, which means clipping them straight across and evenly, then using a nail file to carefully eliminate any pointed ends. If you round the ends, round very minimally. That's it for the dos. Now the don'ts: Don't cut lower than the fleshy part of your toe or into the corners, and don't dig into the toe or along the groove of the nail fold. These are exceptionally tender patches of skin, and you will be happier in life for having left them untouched by anything as sharp as a clipper blade or file edge.

At-Home Treatment of Ingrown Toenails

Caught early, an ingrown toenail can be effectively treated at home by nightly soaking of the feet so that the flesh around the nail remains soft and nonresistant to nail growth. To prevent infection, apply an over-the-counter topical antibiotic ointment such as polysporin or bacitracin to the nail. However, if the area around the nail does not respond to soaking and becomes very painful or red, you should see a podiatrist or dermatologist for treatment. You may need stronger prescribed antibiotics to combat inflammation and ward off infection, or minor office surgery to remove a deeply embedded nail.

Other Common Foot Problems

A sharp-looking pedicure can be a real beauty bonus, especially during the spring and summer months, when most of us show a little toe from time to time. But even nicely pedicured toes won't count for much if they belong to a pair of rough, callused, or foul-smelling feet. If anything, well-groomed nails will only highlight the sad state of a foot (or two!) that could use a dose of tender loving care.

The feet are susceptible to all kinds of minor problems because they take a real pounding. In a lifetime, the average person walks an astounding 115,000 miles, or the equivalent of circling the earth five times. Each of those steps results in the transfer of thousands of pounds of pressure from the body to the feet. Not surprisingly, as many as five layers of skin build up at the soles of the feet to help cushion the shock. Since the soles have no oil glands, those layers of built-up skin are prone to excessive dryness, chapping, and general roughness. In addition, our feet spend nearly every waking hour in the dark, cramped, humid environment created by our hosiery and footwear. Mix in a little perspiration, and you wind up with an ideal setting for the development and reproduction of fungi and

Below:
A fungal infection can occur in either your fingernails or toenails, but toenails are much harder to treat because they are rarely exposed to air. Consult your dermatologist for treatment.

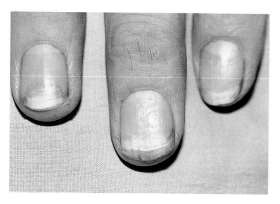

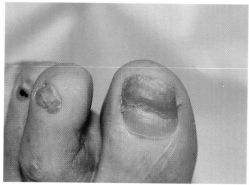

bacteria. Let's run through some of the more common foot problems and see what can be done to (a) keep them from occurring,
and (b) treat them at home when preventive measures fail.

Fungal Infections

Problem: Fungal infections of the toes, toenails, or fingernails
afflict 85% of the U.S. population, though most of
us don't understand the true nature of the problem
when it crops up. Signs of fungal infection include:

- itchy toes
- toenail discoloration
- thick and/or brittle toenails
- separation of the toenail from the nail bed

You are likely to contract a fungal infection—such as athlete's
foot—from not wearing socks, especially during athletic activities or when using a public shower. A sweaty foot in the hot-
house atmosphere of your shoe invites dirt and fungi to waltz in
and multiply at will.

Prevention: To prevent fungal infections, you should always
wear socks—particularly when playing sports—
and wash your feet daily with soap and water.
When washing, be thorough about cleaning and
drying the bottom of the toes and between the toes.
These sheltered, easy-to-miss areas often harbor
the germs that spark fungal infections.

At-Home Treatment: Use a non-prescription fungicidal cream,
lotion, powder or spray such as Micatin™ or
Zeasorb AF™ to combat the infection. If itchiness or
flakiness persist after a week of at-home treatment,
see your dermatologist for something stronger.

Blisters

Problem: Blisters on the feet generally develop as a result of
poorly fitting shoes or socks, both of which create
excessive friction and perspiration.

Prevention: Wear shoes and socks that fit well. Shoes that fit
properly should not pinch or cramp your foot at
any point, yet should be snug enough that your
foot doesn't slide forward when you walk or come

to an abrupt halt. Be sensitive to the width of your shoes (not just the length), and if you err, err on the side of a fit that's too loose as opposed to one that's too tight. Another good tip is to run your hand carefully along the interior of any shoe you wish to purchase: Heavily stitched seams, elastic bands, and rough spots have the potential to rub your feet the wrong way . . . and raise painful blisters! Finally, it never hurts to apply moisturizer to your feet before slipping on your socks. You'll reduce friction that way, plus add needed moisture to one of the driest areas of your skin's surface.

At-Home Treatment: Soak the affected foot in tepid water (or a mixture of soap and water), then pat dry. Next, apply antibiotic ointment to the blister and bandage the wound until it heals completely. NOTE: You should *never pop a blister, under any circumstances.* This invites bacteria into the wound, and can easily lead to a really nasty infection.

Corns & Calluses

Problem: Corns are among the most common foot ailments. They develop on the upper portion of the foot, as well as on top of or in between the toes. An individual corn typically appears as a small patch of thick, callused skin that has become embedded in the healthy skin around it, forming a sort of divot that grows larger, deeper, and more painful as the condition worsens. "Hard" corns generally emerge atop the outside of the small toe; "soft" corns are usually found in the space between the fourth and fifth toe.

Calluses, in contrast to corns, almost always form on the bottom of the foot, and hardly ever cause any noteworthy pain. They appear as patches of thick, roughly textured skin, and can be found most often on the underside of the big and small toes, the heel, and the ball of the foot, mainly because these areas suffer most from the grinding effects of walking (e.g., starting, stopping, turning).

Prevention: Ill-fitting footwear is the main cause of both corns and calluses, so once again, choose your shoes carefully, and always check for rough spots inside. In some cases, rough spots can be padded; in others, the shoes will need to be discarded. Also, vary the height of the heels you wear, to distribute the stress and friction of walking to different points on the ball of the foot.

At-Home Treatment: Soak your feet in warm water until the corn or callus softens, then gently rub the area with a pumice stone or callus file. It will probably take more than one soaking to remove all the dead skin, so be patient and don't go crazy with your stone or file. In between soakings, apply moisturizer to the affected area and cover it with a moleskin or foam-rubber pad to lessen any discomfort that occurs when you're wearing shoes—especially if your job requires you to be on your feet for an extended period.

Some don'ts: Don't attempt to cut off corns or calluses yourself. If things are that far gone, see a podiatrist for professional treatment. Also, don't resort to over-the-counter chemical corn removers or medicated corn pads. They contain acids that eat away the corn—and your healthy skin as well!

Do You "Talk" With Your Hands?

Then all the more reason to ensure that your fingernails always look their best! And even if you don't gesture much during conversation, your hands are probably noticed by others far more often than you imagine. The hands, you see, are front and center in almost every type of social interaction: We shake hands when introduced to new people, hold hands with those we care about, clap our hands to applaud a stirring performance, and display the hands prominently every time we pick up a glass or utensil at the dinner table. For further proof, look to everyday

PRODUCT SPOTLIGHT

Moisturizers for the Hands & Feet

In stark contrast to nearly every other region of the body, the skin on the palms of our hands and the soles of our feet lacks oil glands entirely. Consequently, these areas are prone to dryness, roughness, and chapping, as are the hands and feet in general. To keep your extremities soft, smooth, and supple, it's essential to add back moisture every day. Here are a few products that we have found to be particularly good for the task:

- For the hands, Neutrogena Hand Creme is hard to top. Though the product seems expensive on a per ounce basis, it's really a good value since just a dab of the densely concentrated formula pours moisture back into the skin instantly, rendering hands soft and smooth for the balance of the day.

- For the feet, we recommend Neutrogena Foot Cream, a thick, glycerin-enriched moisturizer that not only softens rough, dry feet almost immediately, but also lasts up to 17 hours per application.

- For care that works while you snooze, try Qtica Overnight Foot Repair and Hand Repair Balms, a pair of thick, rich creams that provide soothing relief for severely dry, sore, and/or irritated skin by effectively sloughing dead cells from the skin's surface and thereby maximizing moisture levels. Both formulations, by the way, are dermatologist-tested and hypoallergenic. Available in beauty salons or by calling Art of Beauty, at 1-800-659-6909.

language—as when you meet the person of your dreams, and are said to "take their hand" in marriage; or help someone in need, and thereby "give them a hand." So whether you "talk" with your hands or not, your hands surely make a statement about you. Take care of them well, and they'll say all the right things!

END NOTES

1. In similar fashion, you'll recall from Chapter Five that a hair shaft derives most of its strength from the *sulfur* bonds that help hold it together.
2. The nails and hair, in fact, continue to grow for a short time even after death.
3. Diet does, however, play a crucial role in the overall health of your skin, as you'll see in Chapter Eight.
4. Nail polishes of all colors contain enamels that typically form a very effective barrier against pigment seepage. For some reason, the pigment in darker shades seem to leech through these enamels occasionally, whereas the pigment in lighter shades almost never does.
5. Nicotine stains from cigarette smoking and exposure to certain hair dyes can also cause temporary yellowing of the nails, and can be treated in the same fashion. If you smoke, though, be aware that frequent, repeated scouring of nicotine-stained nails will ultimately create more problems than it solves.
6. Acrylic polymers are plastic-like substances in liquid form.

For more information on nails, go to *www.apma.org/topics/nail.htm*

NOTES

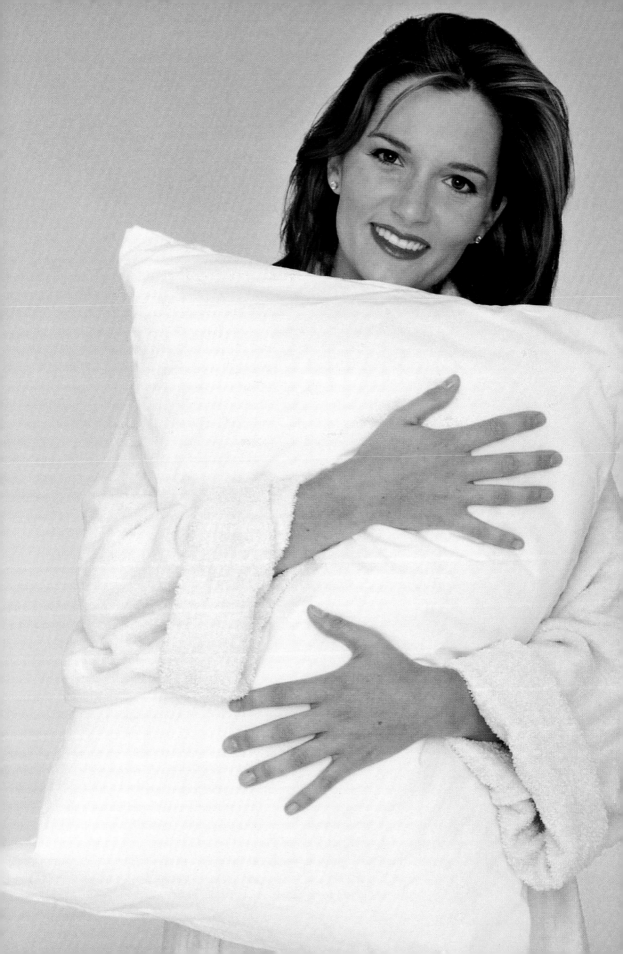

Live Smart, Look Smart: Diet, Exercise, Stress, & Rest

Every day, you make dozens of seemingly innocent decisions that can affect the health and appearance of your skin to a significant degree. At the moment you make them, these may not seem like skin care decisions at all. For instance: Did you miss breakfast this morning? Then have a super-sized burger, fries, and soda for lunch? Did you cut your sleep an hour and a half last night in order to cram for a mid-term? Or skip your aerobics class because you simply weren't in the mood? Or further: Do you dwell on your problems? Constantly worry? Or fret and stew over things beyond your control?

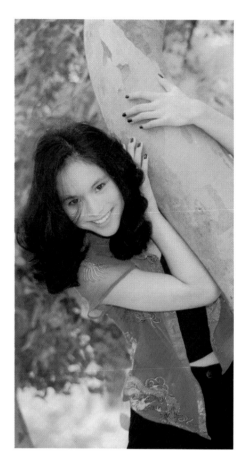

Such decisions and lifestyle choices—along with countless others that affect your general health and wellness—will ultimately be reflected in the color, cast, and overall vitality of your complexion. How could it be otherwise, given that the skin is not only the body's largest organ, but it relies on your internal organ systems for the delivery of oxygen and essential nutrients, as well as the disposal of harmful waste products?

In most cases, the results of hard living—or healthy living, for that matter—are not likely to be directly or immediately apparent, especially now during your teenage years. But they will appear eventually, and their long-term impact can be quite dramatic. Of that much, you can be sure. For proof, look no further than the nicotine-stained fingers and creased mouth of a longtime smoker, or the red, swollen nose of a middle-aged drinker, or the permanently haggard appearance of someone who never, ever seems to get enough sleep. Are you an on-again, off-again dieter? Then watch out! The constant fluctuations in weight you're undergoing may someday become permanently etched into the skin in the form of unsightly stretch marks. Certain diseases, chronic medical conditions, and dietary deficiencies can leave their mark on the skin as well—sometimes temporarily, as with the yellowing of the skin that accompanies a minor episode of jaundice; sometimes for keeps, as with the recurring bouts of increased freckles that characterize a serious case of sun exposure.

We could give more examples, but the basic message is this: Your skin is the terminal point and outward expression of everything that has happened (and is happening) inside you. It follows that a lifestyle that promotes and sustains good health also provides, as a bonus of sorts, the foundation for great-looking skin. In this chapter we will investigate how the lifestyle choices you make today can affect, for better or worse, the way you look tomorrow. Since we are neither dieticians nor psychologists nor experts on sleep or fitness, our discussion is limited to the most basic elements of proper diet, sensible exercise, adequate rest, stress reduction, and the like. We offer some general advice and specific suggestions on each topic, much of which you have no doubt heard before from other sources, but all of which is important enough to be worthy of repetition here. These are, after all, the building blocks of both your health and your appearance, two of the most prized possessions you will ever enjoy!

While we cannot claim expertise in any single area covered in this chapter, we hope that the discussion will reinforce what you already know about healthy living, teach you a few new things, clarify some old misconceptions, and most important, inspire you to learn more about the health and lifestyle issues that are most interesting and relevant to you. First up on our agenda is the much debated, but often misunderstood, subject of diet.

A QUESTION OF PERCEPTION: WHAT DOES "DIET" MEAN TO YOU?

Quick: When you hear the word "diet," do you think instantly of eating—what you eat and how you eat? Or of abstinence from eating—as in cutting your caloric intake or denying yourself certain foods? The question is worth asking, because too many young women, particularly in the U.S., view their diet as little more than a mechanism for weight control. But diet, properly understood, is much more than that. Food is the fuel that keeps us cooking on a cellular level. Consequently, the way we eat has direct bearing not only on those dreaded digits displayed on the electronic scale, but also on our strength, stamina, alertness, longevity, and ability to ward off disease. Too much emphasis on the weight-reduction aspect of diet, we believe, obscures the more significant and positive role that food plays in maintaining optimal health.

If people nowadays appear more fixated than ever on dieting (as opposed to diet), the reason can be at least partially attributed to the glut of new and often conflicting nutritional information we are constantly exposed to. Related to this trend is the steady stream of fad diets that continually find their way into the popular press, each of which seems to capture the public's imagination for a brief period, only to be replaced by a new and, we are assured, better program. One guru tells us we will thrive on a diet consisting mainly of protein, while another points out the various virtues of juices. Some experts say that red meat is OK if you choose the right cuts and downsize the portions, while others adopt a strictly vegan approach. Some folks swear by supplements; others wouldn't touch 'em for love nor money. And on. And on. And on…

Thankfully, the *reality* of eating right is far less complicated than the *hype* of eating right. In a simpler day and time, Home Ec teachers taught their students that there were four main food groups:

- The meat group, which includes not only red meats, white meats, and seafood, but also tofu and nuts (and peanut butter), which typically contain plant proteins
- The dairy group, which consists of milk, eggs, yogurt, and cheese, as well as variations on these animal by-products such as ice cream, sour cream, and cottage cheese
- Vegetables and fruits
- Breads, cereals, and pastas

Although most dieticians now use the food pyramid as a model and make finer distinctions than are reflected in the list above, the four food groups still provide a snapshot of a sensible, balanced diet that contains everything you need for robust health, and in the case of young people, for vigorous growth and development as well. The recommended percentage of your diet that you derive from each group will vary of course, but no one group is more or less important to your health than another. Proteins, carbohydrates, vitamins, certain minerals, and yes, even those much maligned fats, all deserve a place on your plate each and every day.

You might be surprised to learn that the typical American's diet does, in fact, contain generous contributions from each of the major food groups. As a result, the diseases associated with malnutrition[1] don't pose much of a threat for the great majority of U.S. citizens. There are, of course, important exceptions—notably, among the poverty stricken, the homeless, and people suffering from severe eating disorders—but they are seen in a comparatively small percentage of the total population. Our problems, when they occur, more often revolve around the number and type of calories we consume rather than the utter lack of necessary nutrients. Collectively, we often eat too much. And even more frequently, we eat too many of the wrong things. To give just one telling example: Dieticians and other health experts recommend that fats comprise no more than 25% to 30% of our daily diet; yet the average American receives a whopping 40% of calories from fat sources. That fact—coupled with our fast-paced, go-getter society—goes a long way toward explaining why heart surgeons in this country don't have any trouble staying busy! On the other hand, most of us don't eat nearly enough leafy greens, drink enough water, or consume the amount of dietary fiber required for optimal health.

SHAPING A HEALTHY DIET WITH THE FOOD GUIDE PYRAMID

The Food Guide Pyramid, developed by the U.S. Department of Agriculture, expands and refines the traditional concept of the

Below:

The food guide pyramid. (Source: U.S. Department of Agriculture and U.S. Department of Health and Human Services)

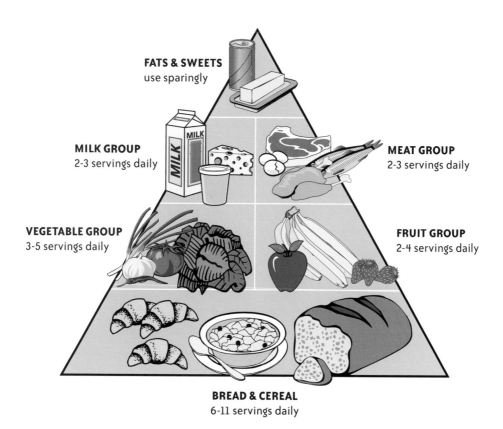

FATS & SWEETS
use sparingly

MILK GROUP
2-3 servings daily

MEAT GROUP
2-3 servings daily

VEGETABLE GROUP
3-5 servings daily

FRUIT GROUP
2-4 servings daily

BREAD & CEREAL
6-11 servings daily

four food groups by clumping meat, fish, and dairy products under the umbrella of protein sources; treating fats and sweets as a separate dietary element; and, most important, revising previously accepted notions about the number of servings that ought to be derived from each group. The illustration on this page tells the story in a very graphic manner, and the key points in that story are pretty simple:

1. Eat more starches.
Starches, which can be derived from whole-grain breads, cereals, rice, and pasta, should serve as the foundation of your healthful, balanced diet. You want to have six to eleven servings from this group on a daily basis. In many foods, including those mentioned above, starches combine with simple sugars (sucrose and glucose are two you may have heard of) and cellulose to form chemical compounds known as *complex carbohydrates*. The beauty of carbohydrates—and the reason so many endurance athletes "load up" on them—is that they are digested easily, burn cleanly, and convert readily into usable energy. An excellent source of dietary fiber, carbohydrates help flush impurities from your system and thus lower your risk of developing intestinal tract cancers and digestive disorders of all kinds.

Below:
Proteins are the building blocks of a strong, flexible body.

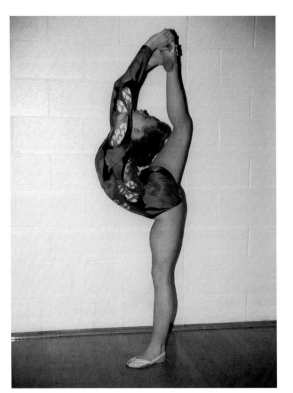

2. Eat more vegetables and fruits.
Fresh produce should also be a prominent part of just about every meal you eat and, as we'll recommend a little later, of your snacks as well. The experts say you need at least five servings daily from this group, but we'd advise that you shoot for the high end of the suggested range (i.e., up to nine servings). Why? Because fresh fruits and veggies are, on the whole, nutrient-dense, meaning they are naturally low in fat and calories, yet rich in essential vitamins and fiber. Recent evidence

suggests, too, that the antioxidant vitamins (A and C) found in fresh produce may dramatically reduce the cancer risk in people who consistently meet or exceed the suggested five serving minimum.[2]

3. Get the protein your growing body needs.
Proteins derived from meats, fish, dairy products, dried beans, nuts, and soy products such as tofu are the building blocks of strong muscles, dense bones, and tough connective tissue. They also play a critical role in repairing damaged muscle tissue when you suffer an injury or strain. In contrast to starches, proteins burn slowly, and act less like fuel and more like raw material once inside your body. Since proteins are especially important for growing adolescents and teens, and for women in general, you should be sure to get your recommended four to six daily servings from this group. For the average American, however, that's no problem. Fact is, our rich diets and hearty eating habits typically provide more protein than we really need, a situation that is further complicated by the fact that much of our protein intake comes from high-fat sources like red meats and dairy products.

Some solutions: Gravitate to low-fat protein sources such as chicken and fish (baked or broiled, not fried!), light dairy products, skim milk, and trimmed, lean meats. Further, slash the fat content of protein sources by thoughtful preparation. It doesn't require much extra effort to, say, remove the skin from the piece of chicken you're preparing or to carefully trim the excess fat from a pork tenderloin before you cook it, yet both of these simple steps can help transform potentially fatty, high-cal dishes into lighter, healthier protein **power** meals.

4. Keep your consumption of fats and sweets to a minimum.
No, we don't expect you to be a nutritional saint here, but fats, oils, and sugars account for untold empty calories in far too many diets. We have already noted that fats make up an excessively high 40% of the average American's diet, and contribute greatly to the incidence of coronary disease in this country. So where does it all come from? From several sources actually, some obvious, some not. Among the obvious offenders we may include rich dairy products, most red meats, most pork, skin-on

chicken, smoked meats, most snack foods (salty or sweet), and fried foods in general. Perhaps the worst of the worst in this category is the stuff you buy at fast-food restaurants, most of which comes packed with fat and calories, yet does next to nothing in terms of satisfying your nutritional needs. Less obvious, but equally disruptive to your dietary balance, are the "hidden" fats that can be found in many canned, packaged, and frozen foods, including such apparently healthy items as pastas, soups, and meatless chilis. Fortunately, tough new laws have forced packaged food manufacturers to provide detailed information about what goes into their products, and stricter standards have been established for the use of common nutritional claims such as "low cal," "lite," "reduced fat," and "high fiber." These new labels are a real plus for consumers. They offer the facts you need to make intelligent nutritional decisions, and should be read religiously by anyone who is at all health-conscious (**see inset box on this page for pointers on what to look for**).

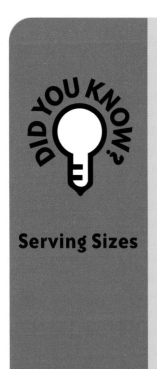

DID YOU KNOW?

Serving Sizes

What you call a serving and what the USDA (United States Department of Agriculture) calls a serving might look very different if placed side by side on separate plates. Yet any difference that exists is important because food manufacturers often base their nutritional information on USDA standards. Let's say you're in the mood for some French fries. You know they're not the most healthful thing in the world, but what the heck, you've been good lately and you've promised yourself that you won't eat more than one 120-calorie serving (a number you've picked up from the side of the freezer bag). If you're like us, you've never in your life actually counted out the number of frozen fries you wanted to eat before placing them on a cookie sheet and popping them into the oven. You've either eyeballed it and used part of the package or simply prepared the whole works. Now, how many fries will wind up on your plate and in your tummy? Our guess is that it will be something more than the ten (yes, 10!) fries that the USDA defines as a single serving. As a result, any casual assumptions you may have made about the number of calories (or the amount of fat and sodium) in your snack were probably way off base.

Listed below are some sample single-serving sizes as defined by the USDA. We've tried to choose relatively common foods, to give you an idea of the gap—if any—that exists between the portions you typically eat and the portions that constitute a serving for labeling purposes.

Item	USDA Serving
Bread	1 slice
Cooked rice, pasta, or cereal	½ cup
Pancakes	1 (4 inches in diameter)
Doughnut or danish	½ medium sized
Cookies	2 medium sized
Vegetables	½ cup
Potato salad	½ cup
Fruits	1 piece, medium sized
Melons	1 wedge
Milk or yogurt	1 cup
Fresh cheeses	1½ ounces
Processed cheeses	2 ounces
Ice cream	1½ cups
Lean beef	2½ to 3 ounces (after cooking)
Fish or poultry	2½ to 3 ounces (after cooking)
Peanut butter	2 tablespoons

Now that you've scanned this list, here are some questions to ponder: When was the last time you ate *half* a doughnut or danish? If a restaurant served you a 2½-ounce cut of meat, wouldn't you wonder where the other half of your entree had gone? What would you like on your (singular) 4-inch pancake? A thimbleful of syrup, perhaps? On a serious note, though, it's important to understand that hearty American-sized servings are often two, three, and four times the USDA definition of a serving. You'll want to take this into account when you shop, cook, and eat out.

As a final note on the fat front, we encourage you to be attentive not only to the foods you purchase, prepare, and eat, but also to the goodies you add to them. A big bowl of rich vanilla ice cream, for instance, is already chock full of calories and fat. But when you immerse it in a river of thick butterscotch topping, the numbers go straight through the roof. Think, too, about the cooking oils, sauces, and salad dressings you choose. These can also sabotage an otherwise well-planned meal. When frying, opt for vegetable oils (canola and olive oil are both good) as opposed to lard, shortening, butter, stick margarine, palm kernel oil, or coconut oil, all of which tend to be high in saturated fat and cholesterol.[3] When making or selecting sauces, find light, low-fat alternatives to the heavy cream sauces, red meat sauces, and gravies your mother used to make. Stock-based sauces, as a rule, are lighter and healthier. The same principles apply to salad dressings, too. The classic olive oil and vinegar combination served in many Italian restaurants, for example, is far better for you than a goopy, high-fat, high-calorie ranch or blue cheese dressing. In general, the thicker and creamier the dressing, the more fat it contains. But do check labels: If the specific type or brand of dressing you prefer is high in fat, you can probably find a lower fat replacement for it if you look around some.

HAVE YOU READ A GOOD LABEL LATELY?

We admit it: Reading food labels is a tedious task. But it's also one of the most important steps you can take toward achieving

Jé Mari's™
(pronounced Jay Maree's)
...the delightfully delicious nonfat frozen dessert!

Jé Mari's™
is a unique blend of the finest and freshest ingredients producing an exceptional rich and creamy texture that tastes like gourmet ice cream. Over **50** scrumptious flavors including Fudge Brownie, Black Raspberry, Caramel Cream and White Chocolate Macadamia Nut... just to name a few!

Jé Mari's™
is naturally sweetened with fruit fructose (no sucrose). Only **10 Fat Free calories** per ounce with **no** cholesterol and **low** lactose!

Satisfy yourself with the *Great Taste* of...

Jé Mari's™

Inside 1 Ounce* of Jé Mari's™	
Calories.....................10	Calcium.....................25mg
Fat 0	Carbohydrates.............3gm
Cholesterol 0	Protein 5gm
Lactose 0.8gm	Sodium 0.04gm

*At 60% Overrun   (KD) Kosher

Jé Mari's™ is made from pure crystalline fructose (fruit fructose), extra grade whey, whey protein concentrate (reduced lactose whey), polydextrose, yogurt solids, natural gums, natural and artificial flavors, and natural colors.

Jé Mari's™ can be enjoyed by most diabetics and lactose intolerants.

Jé Mari's

Mission Viejo • California • USA

a healthy, balanced diet. Here's a quick primer on what to look for as you scan the information on the multitude of bottles, bags, cans, and boxes that fill the typical household fridge or kitchen pantry.

1. *Serving size:* Check the serving size to make sure that it jibes with the portions you ordinarily eat. If it doesn't, you'll need to mentally adjust the other nutritional figures up or down to bring them in line with your dining practices.

2. *Calories from fat:* This tells you how many of the total per-serving calories come from fat. To calculate the percentage of fat in the product, take the calories from fat and divide by the calories per serving. Ideally, the result should be 3% (= .03) or less.

3. *Total fat:* Gives you the number of grams of fat (per serving) the product contains. One gram of fat, by the way, equals nine calories, and you want less than 25% to 30% of your daily caloric intake to come from fat sources. When reading labels, you should get into the habit of asking yourself this question: How close does this product, by itself, bring me to my daily limit for fat? You'll find that some items can actually take you up to—and even beyond—half your daily quota in a single serving!

4. *Saturated fat:* This is a subset of the total fat number; the lower it is, the better. As we saw in our discussion of cooking oils, saturated fats are big-time heart stoppers, so you want to minimize them in your diet.

These are the main items to be wary of, though you should also keep an eye out for excessive amounts of sodium and sugar, too. On the positive side, look for products that post high numbers in the "% Daily Value" column for dietary fiber, carbohydrates, protein, essential vitamins, and minerals like calcium and iron. In most cases, if the fat numbers are low, the nutrient numbers will be high. After all, the calories in the product have to come from somewhere!

SMART SNACKING

Snacking, if you're not careful, can slowly and silently sidetrack your resolutions, damage your health, and expand your waist-

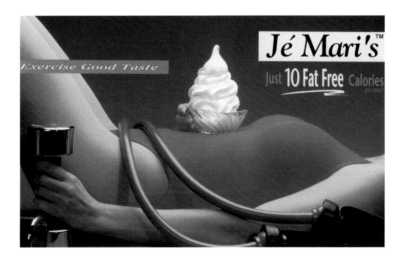

line. Regrettably, candy bars, ice cream, chips, nuts, and other treats too numerous to mention are as much a part of the American dietary landscape as the Rocky Mountains are of the natural landscape. We eat them almost subconsciously throughout the day and into the night—between meals, at work, watching TV, even while we drive. And though no single snacking episode may strike us as especially unhealthful, the cumulative effect of all this constant munching and crunching eventually shows up both inside and outside the body, contributing greatly to the weight problems and heart ailments that currently plague literally millions of us. You may think: "The odd candy bar every now and again won't kill me!" To which we reply: "No, an occasional candy bar probably won't do you in, but a single 2-ounce Snickers does contain 30% more calories and 3 times the fat of *two* comparably sized, fruit-filled granola bars that offer a lot more by way of nutrients and fiber." But even at that, a treat from time to time isn't what ruins most diets. Larger problems arise when your urge to indulge in junk food becomes habitual—when unhealthful snacks start to make up a greater proportion of your daily diet than the lighter, healthier fare you should be eating.

In the real world, of course, our busy lifestyles don't always allow us to eat as regularly and as thoughtfully as we'd like to. In the real world: SNACK HAPPENS. Snacks, however, don't necessarily have to come in a plastic bag or a cellophane wrapper to be quick, convenient, and satisfying. In fact, healthful, natural substitutes for the sweet treats and crunchy goodies you're devouring now can be found throughout the produce section of your neighborhood supermarket. Instead of having a bag of salty corn chips while you catch tonight's episode of fun & romance, why not try crisp carrot and celery sticks with a nice, low-fat dip? When your sweet tooth cries out for chocolate, why not attempt to satisfy the craving with some plump, juicy grapes, a serving of fresh-cut melon, or a bowl of ripe strawberries? All are tasty, nutritious alternatives to the high-cal, high-fat junk food found not only in vending machines but also in most home pantries. Bananas, oranges, apples, pears, and a host of other fresh fruits and veggies also make great go-any-where, eat-anytime snacks. Use them to turn your formerly unhealthy snack attacks into the wholesome, nutrient-rich "mini-meals" that more and more dieticians are recommending as the optimal way to eat!

Before we leave this subject, we should mention that smart snack alternatives can be found outside the produce section, too. Examples include:

- Nonfat frozen yogurt, sorbet, or juice bars as a substitute for ice cream
- Unsalted pretzels, microwave popcorn, rice cakes, or whole-grain crackers as a substitute for potato chips, nuts, and other salty snacks
- Bagels or low-fat bran muffins as a replacement for doughnuts, danish, snack cakes, and other sugary dessert or breakfast treats
- High-fiber fruit bars as a replacement for candy bars
- All-natural fruit juices or flavored waters as an alternative to soda or caffeinated teas

It's Midnight . . .

and you should probably be curled up in bed getting your beauty rest. But instead, you're camped in front of an open refrigerator door, trying to choose between the three remaining slices of last night's pepperoni pizza and a dish of chocolate chip ice cream. Though we confess we've done the same too many times to recall, the fact is that late-night snacks and meals are a real diet "don't." You see, your metabolism slows down as the evening progresses, which means that nearly all of those after-hours calories will tend to go straight to the places you want them least—namely, the hips, buttocks, and thighs. Sweet dreams!

VITAMINS: WHAT YOU NEED, HOW TO GET THEM

In addition to starches, proteins and a modest percentage of fats, your balanced diet must also feature an assortment of key vitamins. Vitamins are complex organic substances that help your body accomplish the metabolic processes necessary to good health. Vitamin K_1, for example, promotes the clotting of blood when you have a cut, and other vitamins perform such unglamorous (but nonetheless vital!) tasks as fostering the passage of nutrients, oxygen, and waste through the walls of your blood vessels and ensuring that your cells replace themselves on a regular basis. And while it may seem that we have known about vitamins since the beginning of time, the truth of the matter is that they were completely unknown prior to the early 20th century. We are, in fact, still discovering new vitamins, and learning more about the properties of old vitamins every day.

For the purposes of our discussion, vitamins can be separated into two broad categories: water-soluble and fat-soluble. In the first group, we may include vitamins C and B complex; in the second, vitamins A, D, E, and K. The distinction between the two types is crucial: water-soluble vitamins are discharged from our systems quickly through urination and perspiration, and so require daily replenishment; fat-soluble vitamins—which are stored in bodily fats—exit at a much more leisurely pace, and so have the capacity to accumulate over time. As a consequence, you can literally overdose on fat-soluble vitamins like A and D, which have been known to reach toxic levels in people who get too gung-ho in their use (or, more accurately, abuse) of dietary supplements containing them.

A Word About Supplements

Generally speaking, we think it is far healthier, not to mention cheaper, to derive the vitamins and minerals you need from natural food sources than from over-the-counter supplements—an opinion still shared, despite the growing popularity of these products, by most of today's medical community.[4] Though you may not realize it, vitamins and minerals are very potent. They occur in extraordinarily minute quantities in the foods you eat; yet anything close to a balanced diet will provide you with the recommended daily allowance (or RDA) of everything that counts, especially when you consider the large and ever-growing number of common grocery items that are now "fortified" or "enriched" with nutrients of all kinds. What's more, your body absorbs vitamins—as well as important minerals such as iron and calcium—much more efficiently when they are delivered in the form of food.

Supplements, by comparison, are an inefficient and, when misused, potentially harmful means of delivery. Look at it this way: You would be hard pressed to find a better or tastier source of vitamin C than a sweet, juicy orange, or a more productive source of calcium than a humble cup of nonfat yogurt. So why in the world would you pay extra for a supplement that doesn't do the job half as well as the natural option? It sure beats us! But if you feel that your diet is dreadfully deficient in certain nutrients, please keep it simple when you supplement. A good multivitamin, taken once a day, ought to provide more than enough of whatever you might be lacking.

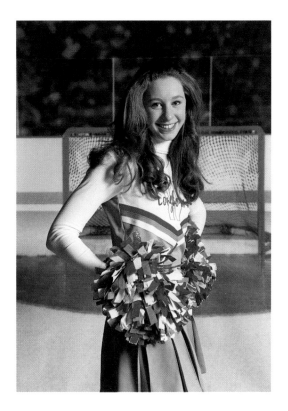

Above:
Three cheers for getting your RDAs, everyday!

A, B, C, D . . . *RDA!*

Although most of us will never experience a serious skin disorder directly linked to the lack of a specific nutrient, vitamins do play an important role in preserving the health and appearance of your skin over the course of a lifetime. Here are five to focus on, along with some good, natural food sources to help you get your RDA of each.

Vitamin A helps foster the proper growth and regeneration of cells throughout the body. As a key element in the cellular replacement cycle, this fat-soluble vitamin is essential to the continuing health of not only your skin but your hair and mucous membranes as well. Specifically, vitamin A promotes skin smoothness and elasticity, which is why it is used in skin care products like Retin-A™. Milk in particular and dairy products in general are often cited as excellent sources of vitamin A (which they are), but you can also derive it from eating fruits and vegetables that are high in beta-carotene, which the body converts into A during the digestive process. Carrots, sweet potatoes, broccoli, spinach, collard greens, canned pumpkin, apricots, and cantaloupe are all excellent nondairy sources of beta-carotene and thus of vitamin A.

Water-soluble **vitamin B complex** is necessary for the maintenance of a smooth, radiant complexion. Conversely, a deficiency in vitamin B complex can lead to scaling and flaking of the skin, as well as dryness and inflammation of the mucous membranes. Brown rice, oats, bran, eggs, yogurt, tuna, chicken, bananas, potatoes, sprouts, broccoli, and dark greens are all healthful, natural sources of this nutrient.

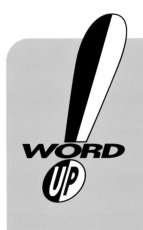

WORD UP

The word "calorie" comes from the Latin *calor*, meaning heat, and is the accepted measure of the energy value of foods. The linkage between food, energy, and heat makes good sense: When we expend energy we generate heat, and thus "burn up" a portion of the calories stored in our body. Calories are therefore as necessary to the proper functioning of the human machine as gasoline is to a car's engine. Neither will run very long without fuel, nor very well without the right kind of fuel. Human beings, to carry the analogy one step further, resemble automobiles in another respect: We come in many different makes and models, each of which consumes fuel at a different rate. Most adult women and nearly all older adults of both sexes constitute the economy models among us, while physically active men and teenage boys can be classified as real gas guzzlers. This last, we are sure, will come as no surprise at all to any reader who has a 16-year-old brother at home!

Vitamin C is an antioxidant vitamin that plays a vital role in the maintenance of blood vessels, the production of collagen, and the healing of wounds. Large doses of vitamin C, consequently, are often recommended for patients recovering from cosmetic surgery. Many experts also believe that vitamin C's antioxidant properties can help keep you looking younger longer by enhancing the skin's ability to fight off certain high-energy molecules known as *free radicals*, which siphon oxygen from healthy cells and thus damage the collagen and elastin fibers essential for maintaining taut, wrinkle-free skin. Citrus fruits and juices, of course, are the best known sources of this water-soluble vitamin, but many other fresh fruits and vegetables contain it, too: These include tomatoes and most varieties of melons on the fruit side; broccoli, Brussels sprouts, and green peppers on the veggie side.

Vitamin D doesn't have a direct connection to skin health, but it is important to the proper development of growing teens. You'll recall from Chapter Three on sun protection that this fat-soluble vitamin is manufactured by the body through routine exposure to UV light. Now, for a fully grown adult who gets outdoors even a little, this internal production alone provides pretty much all the vitamin D he or she needs. Additional quantities of D, however, are required for the formation of strong bones and teeth in both children and teens. To get your RDA, you'll need to drink milk—which here in the U.S. and in most other developed countries has Vitamin D added to it. A couple of glasses a day, plus what you pour on your breakfast cereal in the morning, should just about put you at 100% of the recommended daily allowance.

Like vitamin C, **vitamin E** possesses antioxidant properties, and so may protect your skin from premature aging and wrinkling. A fat-soluble nutrient, vitamin E can be found in wheat germ and sunflower seeds, as well as in several kinds of nuts, including almonds, pecans, and hazelnuts.

The Vitamin Name Game

Many vitamins are identified not only by the letters (A, C, E, B complex, etc.) with which most of us are familiar, but also by biochemical names that often appear on the product labels of packaged foods, skin care items, hair care products, and over-the-counter medications. Here's a sampling:

Vitamin	Also Known As...
A	Retinol[5]
B1	Thiamin
B2	Riboflavin
B complex	Niacin (or nicotinic acid),[6] folic acid[7]
C	Ascorbic acid
E	Tocopherol

The USDA offers these broad guidelines for the total number of daily calories needed to keep us purring along at peak efficiency:

- For most adult women and older adults of both sexes . . . 1,600 calories
- For children, teenage women, active adult women, and most adult men . . . 2,200 calories
- For teenage boys and active adult men . . . 2,800 calories

The daily caloric requirements of any given individual, of course, may vary somewhat from these general guidelines. Your body size and the level of physical activity you engage in, for example, can both move the suggested number up or down. Also, remember from our discussion of the food pyramid that all calories are not created equal: You're much more likely to have lots of pep and vigor if the bulk of your 2,200 calories come from high-octane fuels like whole grain breads, cereals, pastas, and fresh produce as opposed to inefficient sources like fats and sweets. Keep that fact in mind next time you're tempted to "fill your tank" at a fast-food restaurant!

Gross . . . But True!

If you think digestion is a simple process, think again. The human stomach contains an astounding 35 million glands to help break down all the tasty little morsels you send its way. *Juicy!*

Weighing the Pros & Cons of Dieting

Each of us, save perhaps those fortunate few who have all the right pounds in all the right places, possesses some idea of what we would like to weigh. And—at least if our experience is any guide—that "some idea" can be translated into two or three very specific numerals for most teens. (OK, we'll play fair, for most adults, too!) Now, the discrepancy between this ideal weight and our actual weight is often, shall we say, a tad unrealistic—either by virtue of the size of the gap that needs to be covered or by virtue of the complete impracticality of the goal in the first place. But that doesn't stop us from trying! Americans, by and large, are driven by goals and numbers. How much do you make? What's your dress size? Your bust size? Your SAT score? Your GPA? In short, we like to keep score. And even though it adds stress to our lives, we yearn for targets that can be quantified (110 by prom! Size 4 by summer!).

Of course, this kind of goal-oriented behavior does have its good side. When properly channeled, it can help us excel in the classroom, in the workplace, and on the playing field. But it doesn't always work so well when we attempt to apply it to our own metabolism. Sometimes our systems just don't get it, even if we eat the right foods in moderation and exercise with the devotion and intensity of an Olympic athlete. It's worth noting, too, that fewer women strive to gain weight than lose it. If our guess is correct, you've rarely, if ever, had a friend confide over lunch that she was desperately trying to pack on another 12 pounds before swimsuit season, but just couldn't seem to add the weight fast enough. Sadly, weight goals that don't get met almost inevitably lead us to feel as though we have failed to one degree or another. And while many women are able to shrug off this sense of failure quickly and accept their bodies "as-is," a small, yet significant number of us refuse to acknowledge defeat, and become preoccupied with dieting, weight control, and food in general. This is the first step down a slippery slope that all too often culminates in severe eating disorders like anorexia nervosa and bulimia. To avoid taking it, you need to set a realistic weight goal for yourself—one that will allow you to enjoy a full, well-rounded diet that furnishes all the calories and nutrients your body requires for mental alertness, physical stamina, and overall good health. So what's the magic number for you? Let's try to find out!

YOUR IDEAL WEIGHT (WELL, MAYBE)

A rough rule of thumb for determining your ideal weight states that you should weigh about 100 pounds for your first 5 feet in height, plus an additional 5 pounds for every inch above the 5-foot mark.[9] Thus, if you are 5'4" tall your ideal weight, according to this scale, is 120 pounds; if 5'2", 110 pounds; if 5'7", 135 pounds; and so forth. Keep in mind, however, that this is an extremely inexact guideline. While useful perhaps in a very general sense, it assumes that everyone is of identical build, and makes no allowances whatsoever for individual variations in body type, lifestyle (active or sedentary), or metabolism (fast or slow). Yet as we all know, these factors really do matter, sometimes quite a lot. A woman with relatively wide hips, broad shoulders, and thick bones may, for example, tip the scales at 6, 8, even 10 pounds above her so-called ideal weight, yet look slimmer, feel better, and be healthier than a small-framed woman of the same height and lower weight. Muscle mass is another important factor. Muscle weighs more than fat, but looks leaner on the body. So if you've recently started a weight training or resistance program to build mass, what the bathroom scale tells you now may not mean the same thing as it did when you were less muscular.

Ultimately, then, the ideal weight for *you* probably falls somewhere within a fairly broad range, depending mainly on the size and shape of your frame and how muscular (or not!) you happen to be. To illustrate, let's go back to our 5'4" woman. If she is very small framed and sedentary, forget 120—she might not want to weigh more than 112 or 115. If of medium build and reasonably active and fit, then perhaps 120 is just about right. If large framed and muscular, she may feel and look best when in the 125 to 135 pound range. In addition, it's not uncommon for a woman's weight to fluctuate a bit according to the time of day she weighs herself, whether or not she is menstruating, and the amount of water she is retaining at any given moment. We advise you to ignore these minor fluctuations: They really don't tell you anything meaningful about your actual level of fitness or your overall health, and are too often the cause of needless worry and concern.

Some experts, in fact, suggest that there is no such thing as an "ideal" weight, and contend that—even if there were—it would be pointless and unproductive to focus on it. From this perspective, you take care of business by (1) eating a healthy, balanced, low-fat diet; and (2) exercising aerobically on a regular basis. Then, you let your weight find its own level, and ignore the scale. So far, so good, huh? But other equally qualified experts worry that by completely ignoring weight, we also ignore the many health problems associated with obesity, such as excessive stress on the bones and joints, high blood pressure, heightened risk of diabetes, and increased strain on the cardiovascular system. From this perspective, the more weight you carry, the harder your body has to work and the more likely it is to break down prematurely.

Since there is, at present, no definitive answer to this interesting and important debate, it seems to us that drawing positive elements from both points of view is probably the most sensible course of action. For practical purposes, we suggest that you determine your ideal weight as closely as possible by using the scale above and making minor allowances for your size, shape, and lifestyle. Once you've done that, ask yourself a few basic questions, such as:

- Are you reasonably close to your ideal weight? As in horseshoes, close is good enough in the weight game. Wedding yourself to a specific number, as we have seen, can be a recipe for disappointment at best, disaster at worst. Don't go there!

- Do you feel healthy at your present weight? And by this, we mean: Do you have plenty of energy, stamina, and strength? A good (but not insatiable) appetite when meal time comes around? The ability to concentrate when you need and/or want to? If so, then leave well enough alone unless you are more than 20% above the target number or your doctor advises you to lose weight.

- Do you find that you have to practically starve yourself to even approach the ideal weight you've calculated? In this instance, you need to recalculate upward. After all, there's absolutely nothing ideal about an "ideal" weight that renders you sluggish, hungry, and mentally zapped. When that happens, ditch your preconceived notions of what you ought to weigh, and give yourself the nourishment you need. You'll feel—and most likely look—better for it.

Dieting: The Dos, the Don'ts, the Don't You Dares

When you tell a friend that you are about to "go on a diet," the built-in assumption is that there will come a time when you will be "off" that diet. In this sense, a diet is somewhat like a vacation, though perhaps not an altogether pleasant one. You depart for a strange new place, linger a while to see the sights, then return home to the familiar surroundings of your everyday routine. The vast bulk of diets fail, in fact, because the dieter embarks on the new regimen with a short-term weight reduction goal in mind, but has no deep-rooted reason to continue the program once the goal has been reached. Crash dieters are the worst for this. Fully 90% of them eventually regain every ounce they worked so hard to lose—and many regain more. Think about that for a minute: Nine in ten. Scary, isn't it? If a teacher told you during registration that nine of every ten students in her class were going to fail, you wouldn't be in any rush to sign up. Yet thousands of us jump on the diet bandwagon every day—nearly all with good intentions, but remarkably few with a reasonable chance of success.

What demons doom most diets to failure? Let's enumerate:

- **The demon of greed.** If you expect to shed 10 pounds from a 110-pound frame that is already fairly lean, odds are you will find your goal difficult to achieve and almost impossible to maintain. Ten pounds for you is a reduction of more than 9% of your total body weight. To lose that much weight over a 10-week time span (you had figured on a minimum of 10 weeks, hadn't you?) by dieting alone, you'd need to slash your food consumption by 500 calories per day. Unless you're overeating by a wide margin now, that's too much to cut without shorting yourself nutritionally. Remember that 500 calories represents nearly a quarter of the 2,200 daily calories required by the average teenage woman.

- **The demon of speed.** "We want it all, we want it now" could be the mantra of the modern American woman. Unfortunately, what our bodies want most is stability and predictability. You know, that whole "homeostasis" thing from biology class? Short, intense diets run counter to your body's biological urge for equilibrium, and therefore place an incredible degree of stress on your system. What's more, your body can't easily be fooled. It will quickly recognize that it's getting less fuel, and then slow down your metabolism to make more efficient use of the reduced number of available calories. Any weight loss attained in this manner is thus a cinch to be both short-lived and unhealthy.

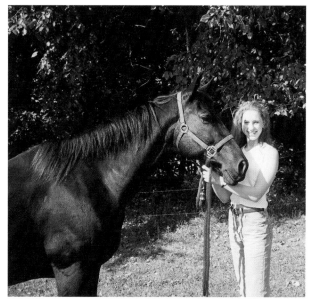

- **The demon of self-denial.** A diet that you view as a form of abstinence or self-denial is highly unlikely to succeed in producing lasting weight loss or a long-term modification of your eating habits. Suffering, while it may seem noble, is actually a very poor motivator, and taste is still the primary reason most of us choose one food over another, despite all the high-sounding talk you hear about nutrition. Consequently, it's naive to think that you will stick to a diet composed of foods you consider bland, tasteless, or downright disagreeable, no matter how badly you may wish to lose weight. To effect a real change, you'll need to go into your new program with a positive outlook and a genuine desire to eat the foods that make up your meals. We've already touched on two relatively easy cures for this common problem: (1) Continue to eat at least some, if not many, of the things you've always enjoyed, but keep the portions modest and

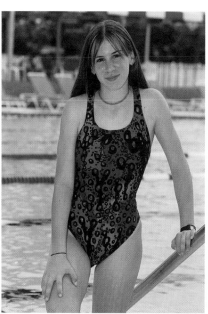

Above:
Sensible eating and plenty of fun activities will keep you fit and healthy.

be careful to avoid adding extra calories or fat through "hidden" sources like sauces and toppings; and (2) replace the worst of your old favorites with similar tasting but more nutritionally sound substitutes.

- **The demon of laziness.** A healthful, low-cal diet, in and of itself, is at best only half the solution to controlling your weight, improving your figure, and optimizing your health. The other half, of course, is exercise. Diet and exercise together form a much more powerful weight-control mechanism than either could on its own, and for this simple reason: When you combine them wisely, you not only enjoy the benefits of taking in fewer calories, but also burn the calories you ingest more quickly and efficiently. Your body, over time, becomes a lean machine that makes the most of every bit of fuel it gets and, as a perk, converts that fuel into firm, shapely muscles and useful energy. Not a bad deal, to our way of thinking.

Characteristics of Diets That Work

How is it that a small percentage of diets succeed long term while most others fail? Offhand, you might think that the willpower of the dieter is a critical factor. Frankly, we don't buy it. In fact, we believe that diets that require willpower to be maintained are flawed from the start. Again, it's not just OK, but positively essential, that you enjoy your food and look forward to your meals. If you find yourself dreading lunch, something has gone wrong! That said, successful diets tend to share some common characteristics. As a rule, such diets are…

- **Based on realistic goals and expectations.** No mystery here, is there? We all know people who, though nicely proportioned or even thin, diet incessantly because they're never quite content with their present weight. Or conversely, we probably also know people who are very overweight, yet get caught in a cycle of on-again, off-again dieting because they seldom persist longer than a few days before relapsing into their old eating habits. In situations like these, the culprit is often an overly ambitious goal. When the target weight is set too low, as in our first example, hunger will generally intervene in a major way and spark a binge of hearty eating that not only effectively ends the current diet but also brings on feelings of failure and guilt. When, as in our second example, the target weight is accurate— but so far removed from present reality as to seem unattainable—the dieter's resolve often crumbles due to the difficulty of the task at hand. Here also, remorse and self-loathing are likely to follow the aborted attempt, and often lead the discouraged dieter right back to the fridge for a dose of that ever-present source of reassurance and comfort called food. Thus the vicious cycle of dieting and overeating perpetuates itself.

So how do you give your weight loss goals a reality check? First, by listening to those around you. If everyone you bump into says you look great or expresses surprise that you're considering a diet, THEY PROBABLY MEAN EVERY WORD. Sure, people like to be nice. But they're not *that* nice. Further, if you're catching lots of comments that you seem too thin or look as though you're not eating enough, that's also probably true. For some reason, suggesting to someone that she is overweight is pretty much taboo in our society, but the politeness doesn't apply in reverse. So if friends and relatives are telling you—if not directly, then in so many words—that you don't need to diet, it's likely that they're right on the money. Our second reality check is perhaps the simplest of all: Look in the mirror before you look at the scale. Numbers that sound big to you may look just fine on your frame, especially if you are tall, or broad through the shoulders and hips. Last, if you have lots of weight to lose, don't intimidate yourself with double-digit goals. Take it a step at a time by establishing very small, achievable, short-term goals. Even if you ultimately hope to slim down by 50 pounds or more, you'll probably get there more surely, less stressfully, and (surprise, surprise!) faster by working a pound or two at a time than by trying to do it all at once. Setbacks are time-consuming and emotionally draining, so don't set yourself up for them. Instead, proceed slowly—then never look back!

• **Gradual.** As we observed earlier, trying to lose too much, too fast can leave you lacking in important nutrients and the energy they provide. As a result, health experts almost universally recommend that you keep your calorie count up to a reasonable level by spreading your desired weight loss over an extended period of time. In practice, that usually means framing your weight loss goals in terms of months, not days or weeks. In the case of a truly obese person, the final weight goal may even be 3, 4, or 5 years distant, with several short-term goals (as we've suggested) along the way to help measure progress and sustain the dieter's motivation. While the "slow but sure" approach admittedly requires some patience, study after study has shown that pounds shed gradually are much more likely to stay off than pounds shed through short, intense bouts of dieting. It's also a more healthful approach, since your system can adapt to the new regimen at a leisurely pace and is spared the shock of a sudden, dramatic plunge in calories. Generally speaking, you shouldn't attempt to lose more than a pound or two per week, no matter how much weight you eventually hope to drop.

• **Sustainable.** This ties in to a pair of points we've already mentioned. First, that you should find foods for your diet that appeal to you; and second, that your diet should be substantial enough to keep you healthy and energetic. Hint: If you experience sharp hunger pangs between meals or late at night, you ought to reassess your diet to make sure that it provides a sufficient number of calories and isn't skewed *too* heavily toward quick-burning carbohydrates. While carbohydrates are great for your overall health and should account for a healthy percentage of your total caloric intake, you cannot and should not let them *dominate* your diet. When that occurs, the dieter often finds that she never feels quite full, and develops an abnormally strong desire for fats and sweets. Not good!

In the end, a diet composed of mostly healthful foods that you enjoy eating—in quantities sufficient to keep your health robust and your appetite satisfied—is the only safe, sane, and lasting solution to any weight control problems you may have. If you can do that, plus keep your portions to a reasonable size, you will have done about as much as you humanly can to regulate your weight through food alone.

"I'm Soooo Skinny..."

For many fast-growing teens, the problem isn't losing weight but adding enough to stay abreast of a rapid rise in height or an exceptionally active metabolism. If this describes you, try not to become too self-conscious, and more important, be careful to avoid the common error of beefing up your diet in an attempt to restore proportion to your frame. In most cases, the "skin and bones" look that makes you feel gawky and awkward today will fill in quite nicely once your growth spurt runs its course, usually as you enter your late teens or early twenties. Hence there is no sense in developing bad eating habits (which may last a lifetime) for what is likely to be a passing occurrence. For now, eat heartily and eat healthfully—and be thankful you can! But don't purposely overindulge. Someday, years from now, you may actually find yourself looking at a picture of your skinny teen self and wishing you could have that thin body back!

EATING DISORDERS: BY THE NUMBERS

Estimates vary as to just how many Americans are currently afflicted with eating disorders. The numbers are difficult to pin down with any degree of accuracy, for a couple of reasons: First, doctors aren't required to provide data on the subject; and second, so many victims either conceal their illness or deny they have a problem at all. Be that as it may, experts in the field offer an educated guess that 8 million of us suffer from anorexia nervosa, bulimia, binge eating, or a related disorder. While a thorough examination of these complex and potentially life-threatening conditions is beyond the scope of our discussion here, you should know at least this much: **90% to 95% of people with eating disorders are women, most of whom range in age from early adolescence to their mid-20s.**

This is YOU, dear reader! Your generation is bearing the brunt of the very real emotional and physical havoc caused by eating disorders. Right now, in fact, you probably have at least one friend, classmate, co-worker, or sibling who is either suffering silently or in denial. So learn all you can—especially about the warning signs—not only for your own sake but also for the sake of the people you care about. A support group called ANRED (short for Anorexia Nervosa and Related Eating Disorders, Inc.) has published a useful questionnaire for just that purpose. It can be found on their website at http://www.anred.com. A similar questionnaire known as the

EAT Test has been developed by researcher and eating-disorder expert David Gardner, Ph.D.[8] Though many of the questions posed in the two documents are nearly identical, Dr. Gardner's test differs from the ANRED quiz in that it assigns numerical values to the test-taker's answers and offers an assessment of risk based on the resulting score.

EXERCISE

Regular exercise is the logical companion to—and complement of—your good eating habits. It not only helps you stay slim and trim, but also builds and tones the muscles, improves bone density, strengthens the cardiovascular system, and increases your capacity to process oxygen. The resulting benefits to your skin, as you might imagine, are many and varied: Toned muscles and strong bones, for example, provide just the sort of framework needed for smooth, firm skin, and enhanced blood flow, for its part, ensures that a plentiful supply of nutrients and oxygen reach all those tiny capillaries that nourish your skin cells from head to toe. Exercise can also reduce stress levels and thus temper the hormonal surges induced by stress, which lessens the likelihood that you will suffer from certain types of hair loss conditions, nail problems, and skin disorders. But last, and most important, an adequate level of physical fitness lays the groundwork for sound overall health, which will be reflected in everything from the color of your complexion to the very texture of your skin.

Aerobic vs. Anaerobic Exercise

Physical activities that condition the body can be split up into two very broad categories: *aerobic* and *anaerobic*. Now, you may have read else-

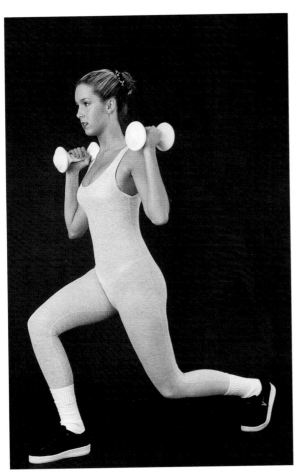

Below:
Weight training is a valuable part of any workout.

where that certain kinds of exercise, such as running, bicycling, stair-stepping, or swimming, are "aerobic." You may even currently participate in an aerobics class. Conversely, you may have heard that weightlifting is an "anaerobic" form of exercise. Now, such distinctions, though generally true based on the way most people exercise most of the time, can nonetheless be misleading. The word aerobic literally means "in the presence of oxygen." Used precisely, it can therefore be applied to any exercise that requires your cardiovascular system to work harder than normal, but not so hard that it fails to keep up with the oxygen needs of the muscles being exercised. By extension, an activity can be accurately labeled as anaerobic when the intensity level of the exercise pushes the working muscles to the point that they require more oxygen than your body can deliver in a timely fashion.

Seen from this perspective, the workout you get in your aerobics class may or may not always be aerobic. If everything proceeds at a smooth, steady pace that doesn't surpass the limits of your current cardiovascular conditioning, then well and good. You're probably exercising aerobically, even if you've worked up a light sweat. But when the music is cranking and you really start to jam, odds are that you will quickly outstrip the capacity of your heart and lungs to send fresh, oxygenated blood to your legs and arms, thus taking the workout to an anaerobic stage. Running also provides a good illustration of our point. When you run at a light jogging clip, as most folks do, the activity is aerobic. But push it to an all-out sprint, and you're definitely in anaerobic territory.

Aerobic Exercise & Heart Health

The distinction between aerobic and anaerobic exercise is important because each delivers different health benefits and improves your conditioning in different ways. Aerobic workouts, on the whole, are best for improving your overall stamina, keeping yourself lean, and strengthening your cardiovascular system; anaerobic workouts are generally best for toning and sculpting the physique, increasing raw strength, and building muscle mass. This being the case, nearly all health experts would encourage you to make aerobic conditioning

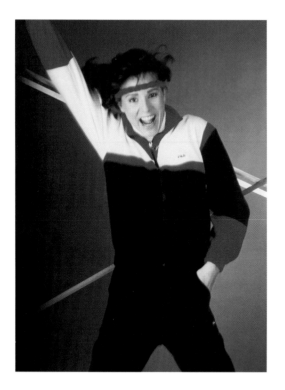

your first priority, then move on to anaerobic (or strength) training later. You see, though all exercise tends to strengthen a specific muscle or group of muscles, aerobic exercise zeroes in on the most important muscle of all—the heart. When you condition yourself aerobically, the walls of your heart actually thicken and the muscle itself becomes more efficient and more powerful, allowing you to do the same amount of work at a lower pulse rate than before. In time, other cardiovascular benefits follow. Your overall blood volume increases, your circulation improves, and new capillaries branch out from existing ones to help transport the now-abundant output of your super-efficient heart.

But Wait . . . There's More!

Of course, aerobic exercise would rank as a health (and beauty!) must on the basis of the above-mentioned benefits alone. But that's not nearly the end of the story. For starters, an aerobically fit body is a body with a high metabolism rate, meaning that it burns more calories during inactive periods and sleep than it would otherwise. A good workout, in fact, will stimulate your metabolism for several hours afterward, causing calories to be consumed at a faster than normal rate long after you've showered and left the gym. In addition, aerobic activity helps clear fats (called triglycerides) from the bloodstream, and promotes a more favorable cholesterol balance[10] in those who exercise regularly. Still not sold? Then consider this: A surprisingly small investment of time and effort in aerobic training will also pay big dividends in the form of leaner, shaplier muscles, better posture and improved resistance to illnesses both minor and major.

Fat Blasters & Calorie Cutters

Recent research conducted at the University of Missouri-Columbia puts jogging at the head of the exercise pack in terms of gobbling up fats, burning calories, and improving cardiovascular health. The study compared several common forms of exercise for these attributes, and yielded the following results:

Most Effective	Jogging (at a comfortable but still challenging pace)
	Ski simulation
	Rowing (on a machine)
	Stationary bicycling or spinning class
Least Effective	Stepping

As you scan these results, bear in mind that all of the listed exercises, as well as some that aren't listed, such as power walking and swimming, provide tremendous heart health and fitness benefits. Though jogging emerged as the clear winner, there really are no losers in this bunch.

Just a Little Exercise Goes a Long Way

Despite the many obvious benefits of exercise, most of us turn the recent Nike advertising slogan straight on its head. In a phrase: WE JUST DON'T DO IT. We spend too much of our time in cars, at desks, in front of the TV, and glued to computer screens, and not nearly enough time in the gym or the great outdoors. Obesity in America has been escalating for many years now, especially among young people, and our increasingly sedentary lifestyle makes a quick turnaround in this trend seem highly unlikely. *You*, however, can buck the trend—and the best part is, it's almost sinfully easy. In fact, **nearly all of the beneficial health effects of aerobic exercise can be derived from just three 30-minute sessions per week.** That's a grand total of 1½ hours weekly, perhaps less time than you often devote to surfing the Internet or watching music videos in a single evening!

If staying in decent shape requires such a minimal commitment, you may ask, then why do so many people fail to get the exercise they need? This is a complex question, and the answers to it are as varied as the legions of well-intentioned individuals who think about starting an exercise program, yet never quite get past the thinking stage. Lack of time is probably the most frequently cited reason, but let's be honest: Who among us is so busy that she can't wedge in a half hour of exercise every other day? A few overburdened souls, perhaps, but not many. Truth is, we either find time or make time for the things we really want to do, so the real reason most exercise resolutions aren't fulfilled is that the people making them aren't motivated enough to get one started and stick with it. Exercise, for many of us, simply seems too much like drudgery—and feels too much like duty—to be viewed in a positive light. That popular word "workout," with its connotations of sweat, toil, and obligation, speaks volumes about prevailing perceptions and attitudes. It's as if we were saying: "This isn't fun. This isn't invigorating. This is work—and hard work at that." Small wonder, then, that so many new jogging suits are more often used for lounging on the couch than for pounding the pavement!

Getting Started Begins With Getting Motivated

We suspect that the widespread perception of exercise as work—at least for many folks—begins at an early age. Too many gym teachers and youth coaches still approach their jobs with a boot camp mentality, and thus use calisthenics, running, and organized sports as a means of whipping their "troops" into shape. Worse yet, some of them even go so far as to use exercise as a form of punishment. This "give me twenty" type of thinking is outdated, wrong-headed, and damaging. In reality, the exercise you do needn't be grueling or forced to be effective. Quite the opposite, as a matter of fact! To succeed in the long run, your exercise regimen—like your diet—should consist primarily of activities you not only enjoy, but actually look forward to. So if water skiing and tennis are your favorite recreational activities, for gosh sake, water ski or play tennis. Don't take up something else simply because it seems more like "real" exercise. Aerobic conditioning occurs when your heart beats at 70% to 80% of its maximum rate for 20 minutes or more. And guess what? Your heart doesn't have the foggiest notion whether you are running on a treadmill, rollerblading, playing basketball, windsurfing, or gyrating like a madwoman to the sounds of a hot new alternative band. All it knows is that it's working harder than normal, though hopefully within a healthy range. Thus, while it's true that a certain amount of self-discipline may be required on days when you are tired or down in the dumps, there really is no substitute for genuinely liking your exercise (or exercises) of choice. Get this part right and you will not only be well on your way to starting a fitness regimen but also to sustaining it for a lifetime.

Six Simple Ways To Stay Injury-Free

In fairness, we must admit that the initial hurdles of starting to exercise, then getting into shape, cannot be overcome without some degree of physical exertion and subsequent muscular discomfort. To that extent, we suppose, exercise really is work, especially if you are currently overweight or happen to be coming off a very low fitness base. And though we definitely do not agree with the "no pain, no gain" school of thought, this post exercise discomfort is a price that must be paid—at least for a while—by anyone who is not already fit, yet would like to become so.

The reason for this is that conditioning takes place on a muscular level through an ongoing process of damage, repair, and rebuilding. When you exercise strenuously but properly, the fibers that compose your working muscles develop slight tears that aren't significant enough to cause real injury but do cause short-term soreness and fatigue. If you've done things right and haven't pushed yourself too far, those torn fibers will mend during the intervals of rest between exercise sessions and, in fact, come back stronger and more resilient than before. In technical terms, this is what is known as the *conditioning effect*. For those who wish to attain an acceptable level of fitness and then simply maintain it, the early discomfort associated with exercise will gradually diminish, and ultimately fade altogether once the muscles have adapted fully to the demands routinely placed on them. But for those who wish to build fitness to optimal levels, the cycle of increasingly strenuous exercise, followed by muscle fatigue and soreness, followed by rest and recovery, will be more or less constant until a level of peak conditioning has been reached.

Since the conditioning effect, of necessity, requires that you push certain muscles to the threshold of their present strength and endurance in order to build or improve fitness, the risk of suffering an injury is always just around the corner. At low levels of muscular stress, such as a short, brisk walk or a brief spin on an exercise bike, this risk is obviously very minimal. You're more likely to injure yourself grievously on a walk by tripping over a sidewalk crack or getting hit by a car, for example, than by anything you'll do by the exercise itself. More arduous activities, though, hold the potential for everything from minor strains and sprains, to serious problems like exercise-induced asthma and even heart failure. We don't say this to scare you, but facts are facts. Anyone who has ever participated in a charity "fun run" has probably signed a form stating that they understand that the health risks of their 3-mile jog in the park include such unsavory possibilities as heart attack, stroke, broken bones, respiratory problems, and death, to mention just a few. That language, friends, is in there because such unpleasant events, though uncommon, actually occur on rare occasions. Fortunately, though, the long-term health benefits of exercise far outweigh the largely avoidable risks that accompany it. To reduce your chances of getting hurt while you're getting fit, we advise that you take a half dozen simple, common-sense precautions:

1. Schedule a complete physical with your family physician before you begin any new exercise program or significantly increase the intensity or frequency of an existing one. In most cases, your doctor will not only give you the medical go-ahead to exercise, but also applaud and support your efforts. But do not make the mistake of taking this step for granted or considering it a mere formality. Many collegiate and professional athletes—in other words, some of the most highly conditioned people in the world—have suffered strokes, had seizures, and even died on the practice field from preexisting conditions that had gone undiagnosed. So get that checkup right away. It's a mandatory first step.

2. Wear appropriate protective gear and clothing. For cyclists, skate-boarders, and rollerbladers, this translates to donning a *helmet, elbow pads, and knee pads,* not just when you feel like it but *every time out*, to help prevent the broken bones, concussions, and serious head injuries of all kinds that occur much more often than most participants in these activities realize. Long pants and a long-sleeved top are also good ideas for prevention of cuts, scrapes, and bruises. Runners and walkers, for their part, will want to choose the right shoes to absorb the shock of the thousands of pounds of pressure that result from each footfall, plus wear reflective clothing when they run or walk at night (ditto for cyclists). Of course, we can't cover every sport here, but you get the drift. Now, get the gear and wear it!

3. Listen to your body. When you overexert, your body almost always gives you advance warning that something bad is about to happen if you don't back off. During exercise, the most serious of such warnings may come in the form of extreme shortness of breath, a galloping pulse, severe muscle cramping, dizziness, or sharp pain of one sort or another. When you get these signals, you need to STOP what you are doing immediately. These are big-time red flags, and you ignore them at your peril. What's more, if one of these signals persists after you've had a chance to rest briefly, don't wait a day to see what happens. Have someone take you to a doctor pronto.

The body delivers subtler messages, too, which nonetheless provide important information to those who understand them. The simplest to monitor are your heart rate and respiratory rate. Many high-tech gadgets now exist to keep tabs on your heart rate electronically, but you can get by just fine without the cumbersome paraphernalia. To check your heart rate during exercise, lightly rest your finger on an artery and count the beats for 10 seconds, then multiply by 6. The result you get should be higher than your normal resting pulse rate (taken before exertion), but it shouldn't be off the charts. A commonly used guideline[11] offers the following formula for determining the "target zone" heart rate for someone who is aerobically fit: (220 − your

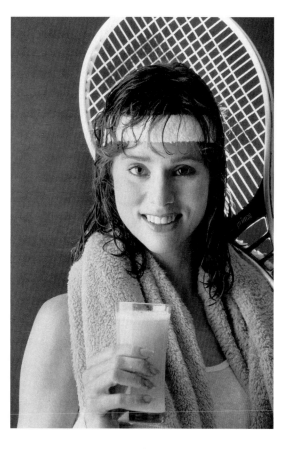

Above:

Be sure to get plenty of fluids before, during, and after exercise to prevent dehydration.

age) $\times$ .7 or .8. For a fit 18-year-old, the math would run this way:

> 220 $-$ 18 $=$ 202 (maximum heart rate during exercise)
>
> 202 $\times$ .7 $=$ 141.4 (or about 141 beats per minute; low end of training range)
>
> 202 $\times$ .8 $=$ 161.6 (or about 162 beats per minute; high end of training range)

For safety's sake, well-conditioned people should try to keep their level of exertion within or below the defined training range pretty much all the time, and should never exceed their maximum heart rate. Beginners, on the other hand, can usually improve their fitness at much lower levels than those listed above, so should not attempt to work out at target zone heart rates until they have successfully completed several months of progressively more demanding aerobic activity.

The test for monitoring your respiratory rate, which is aptly called the "talk test," is even easier to perform than the heart rate test. Simply stated, you should be able to carry on a brief conversation in relative comfort while you're working out. In practice, this means that if you can't reply to a question or talk to the person next to you in your aerobics class without gasping for breath, your body is saying (in a breathless fashion) that you've exceeded the limits of your current conditioning and need to slow down.

Proper hydration is another important factor to keep tabs on while you exercise. But in this particular instance, you are better off *anticipating* your body needs rather than waiting for a signal. Thirst, of course, is your body's way of telling you it wants a drink. However, your system is already somewhat dehydrated by the time you become thirsty, especially during heavy exercise. So it's important to make frequent water breaks a planned part of every workout. Pausing for an instant to take water won't detract from the quality of the workout, and it may even enable you to exercise harder and longer than you would have otherwise. If you participate in endurance sports such as distance running, cycling, or triathlons, you may also wish to alternate the drinking of water with consumption of a specially formulated sports drink like Exceed or Gatorade to replenish the lost electrolytes and nutrients your body burns up during

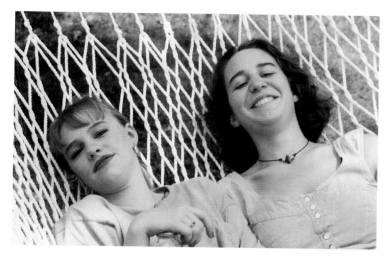

Left:
Take a break! Your body needs a day off from exercise to prevent fatigue and over-use injuries.

strenuous exertion. Start small, though. While many people have no problems with these drinks, others find them upsetting to the stomach if they drink more than a few sips at a time while working out.

4. Include rest in your routine. As you'll recall from our discussion of how muscles (including the heart) become stronger, rest is a necessary component of any exercise regimen. In fact, it takes your muscle fibers about two full days to recover completely from the effects of vigorous exercise. Now, this doesn't mean that you are limited to exercising every third day, or that you have to be completely inactive on your "off" days. A very light, low-impact workout, for instance, qualifies as rest, and may even speed the recovery of exercise-fatigued muscles by causing extra blood to be sent their way. Similarly, an anaerobic training session can count as rest from the previous day's aerobic workout if different muscle groups are used, and vice versa. You should, however, treat yourself to a full day of rest at least once or twice a week, especially if you are the type that tends to get manic about exercise. Too much uninterrupted training can easily lead to overuse injuries, increased susceptibility to cold and flu bugs, and a generalized sense of mental and physical exhaustion, all of which will set your fitness back much farther than the odd day off ever will.

5. Build fitness gradually over time. A fitness routine founded on the idea that you can make up for years—or even months—of inactivity with a short flurry of intense work is mis-

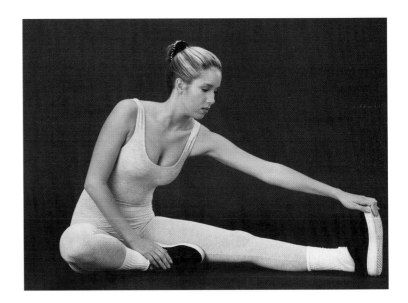

Right:
Always take the time to warm up and cool down with stretches to avoid injury during exercise.

guided at best, downright dangerous at worst. Recall what we said earlier about dietary changes and your body's natural inclination toward equilibrium. Well, the same holds true for exercise. When you try to achieve too much, too quickly, you're fairly begging to get hurt. A safer and more fundamentally sound approach is to progress in small, measured steps from month to month, and also allow yourself time to plateau for a while at each new stage of fitness. While this may seem counterproductive, especially if you tend to be the impatient, goal-driven sort, it's important to realize that *the days and weeks you spend maintaining fitness are every bit as crucial to the long-term success of your program as the days and weeks you spend building it.* You should view them not so much as a delay in progress but as a means of cementing the gains you've made to date.

6. **Warm up before you work out, and cool down after.** A warm-up consisting of 10 to 20 minutes of low-intensity aerobic exercise and light stretching is a necessary but all too often neglected prelude to nearly every kind of prolonged physical exertion, including such seemingly harmless activities as playing a pickup game of sand volleyball or hiking the trails of a nearby park. The purpose of these preliminaries is two fold: first, to gently prepare your cardiovascular and respiratory systems for the work ahead; and second, to warm, loosen, and increase the flexibility of cold, stiff muscles and connective tis-

sue (i.e., tendons and ligaments). The aerobic part of your warm-up—which can be achieved through brisk walking, stationary cycling, or marching in place—should last 5 to 10 minutes, and a comparable amount of time should be devoted to stretching.

When you stretch, concentrate on holding each stretch to a point of mild tension for 8 to 10 seconds; then repeat until the stretched muscle feels nice and limber. Try to cover all of the major muscle groups, but zero in on the areas you intend to exercise. Focus, too, on maintaining proper form. Stretching is best accomplished through slow, smooth movements that gradually elongate the various muscles that will be brought into play during the workout. So don't bounce, don't jerk, and don't be in a hurry. You want to stretch in the same manner as you'd reach for a delicate piece of china on the top shelf of your kitchen cabinet—deliberately, carefully, and with a view toward making yourself as long as possible without losing balance or causing undue strain. Hang on to that mental image, and you will stretch properly more often than not.

Once your workout is complete, cool down by repeating your warm-up routine, but in reverse order. This not only helps prevent your muscles from becoming tight and sore, but also provides a "soft landing" for your body as it transitions from its hyped-up exercise mode to relative inactivity.

What Have You Done for Me Lately?

You've no doubt heard the term "muscle memory" before. It's used to describe the body's almost uncanny ability to repeat and refine learned physical skills such as riding a bike, throwing a softball, or dancing the Macarena. But when it comes to brute exertion, your muscles have a relatively short memory. Perhaps they'd just as soon forget about those weights you made them lift or the grueling cheerleading drills you put them through! In any event, your muscles typically "remember" how hard they've recently worked for a period of about 1 to 2 weeks. As luck would have it, that's just enough time to weather most colds, take an exercise-free vacation with your family, or focus exclusively on schoolwork during finals—without losing much of your hard-earned fitness. But if you shun exercise longer than a couple of weeks, you'll need to build back lost strength before resuming where you left off.

Tired of That Old Ab Machine?

Monotony—and the boredom it engenders—can eventually bring even a well-established exercise regimen to a slow, grinding halt. Yes, an easily amused few can swim (or run, or step, or practice tae-bo) five times a week for years on end and never tire of the activity. But the rest of us need some variety, at least occasionally. So it's smart to mix things up once in a while. To do so, we advise that you take a broad view of exercise and use some creativity in planning your workouts. Let's say you played volleyball throughout junior high, but dropped it during high school because you didn't have the time to practice 3 days a week with the team. Would it be crazy to suggest that you join a church or intramural league that plays only once a week, just for the sake of fitness and fun? Or again: If you love to dance, why not make it a point to go to a club at least once every week or two with someone who's into it as much as you are, then stay on the floor long enough to get a good cardiovascular workout? Even mundane tasks can be the occasion for exercise, provided you keep your mind open to opportunity. Example: If your dog strains at the leash every time you walk her, don't fight it. Go with the flow and aerobicize the event by alternating light jogging with brisk walking. The pooch will think she's croaked and gone to canine heaven, and you'll get a nice workout. Your routine, to sum up, is only as routine as you make it. Get out there and do something new today!

STRESS

Exercise has often been touted—accurately, we might add—as an extremely effective means of relieving stress. And small wonder! Thousands of years of evolution have conditioned our bodies to respond to stress with action. This is so because the earliest human beings lived in a hazardous, terrifying world—one in which only those who reacted swiftly and decisively to the threats around them survived to pass on their genes to later generations. Can you imagine, for example, how stressful your life would be if, like a primitive hunter, you had to take down a huge, aggressive animal with a slender wooden spear or a stone-tipped arrow, then face the prospect of starvation if you failed? Or if your only refuge from the winter cold was a dark, dank cave, which other predators such as bears and wolves might also wish to inhabit? Well, our distant biological ancestors faced these kinds of challenges every day; and from them, we have inherited an elaborate internal alarm system that not only alerts us to menacing situations but also physically prepares us to respond by either combating or fleeing the perceived threat.

Biologists refer to this as the "fight or flight" response, a physiological sequence of events triggered whenever we sense that danger is close at hand. While the threat itself may be genuine (an oncoming car abruptly turns in front of you) or imagined (you mistake a random noise outside your bedroom window for someone trying to break into the house), the response itself is always real. Adrenaline and other hormones quickly flood your system, your pupils dilate, your heartbeat quickens, your blood pressure rises, your blood sugar level escalates, and your muscles contract. Your body, in short, is now primed and pumped to either bonk someone on the head or run the other way with the speed of a freshly launched bottle rocket. But since the threats that confront us today are chiefly emotional or psychological in nature, all of this intense preparation for physical action usually winds up going for naught. We can't, after all, jump up from our desk and run away from a test we're worried about failing—the way primitive man might flee a charging rhino—nor engage in hand-to-hand combat with a rival who constantly flirts with our boyfriend (though the thought may have crossed our mind once or twice).

Instead, our stress tends to become internalized. We keep things inside, and lacking an acceptable means of relief, often

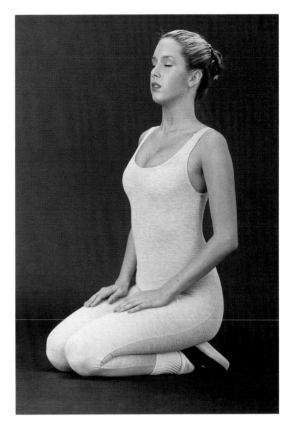

Above:
Yoga is great for relieving stress, increasing flexibility, and using breathing techniques to help you feel "centered."

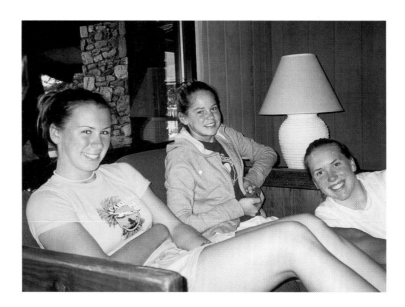

Right:
*Spending time with friends is
a guaranteed stress buster!*

find that the symptoms of stress not only fail to subside but actually feed on themselves and build. When this occurs, our skin responds in a number of ways. Typically, the skin's most immediate response to stress is one with which we are all familiar: Our face becomes flushed, whether we are blushing from embarrassment because of an unexpected compliment, or steaming with rage due to a rude remark. If the stimulus is strong enough, we may even begin to perspire or develop gooseflesh on the spot. More serious skin reactions, which generally result from stress that is either constant or very intense, are possible too. These include hives, warts, hair loss, and eczema, among others. In addition, certain preexisting skin conditions, such as acne and dandruff, can be aggravated by the hormonal imbalances caused by stress.

Though the skin problems associated with severe or unrelenting stress can be significant, the damage to your overall health can be far greater. In fact, the ailments linked to excessive stress range in gravity from disrupted sleep patterns, indigestion, and diarrhea, on the one hand, to serious emotional disturbances, chronic digestive disorders, high blood pressure, and heart disease, on the other. People under heavy stress are also prone to suffer from chest pains, backaches, headaches, and shortness of breath, and often find it difficult to think clearly, act decisively, or control their moods.

How Much Is Too Much?

Since all of us live with some degree of stress nearly every waking moment, it isn't always easy to distinguish normal levels of stress from levels that may be unhealthy. There are, however, many well-documented physical and psychological warning signs that can help you determine if the amount of stress in your life has reached a potentially dangerous point. We've grouped these signs below by type, and suggest that you seek professional treatment if you discover that several items in both categories frequently apply to you.

Physical Signs	Psychological Signs
Difficulty sleeping	Uncontrollable mood swings
Racing heartbeat	Nervousness and irritability
Shortness of breath	Tendency to overreact
Digestive problems	Inability to think clearly,
Headaches	concentrate
Backaches	Lack of decisiveness
Chest pain	Faltering relationships
	Dwelling on problems
	Feelings of entrapment
	or paranoia
	Declining self-esteem

Getting the Best of Stress

So long as stress hasn't assumed control of your life, practical steps can be taken to cope with it, relieve it, and minimize its unpleasant effects. Below, we've offered some stress-busting strategies for you to use, which fall into two groups: Quick tips for immediate relief, and big picture suggestions to help you keep everything in perspective. Since our list isn't nearly exhaustive, we hope you will use it not only for the advice it contains but also as a springboard for developing your own stress-management techniques.

Quick Tips

- Yawn and stretch. It's the body's natural mechanism for relieving pent-up tension.
- On a related note, take a few deep breaths to clear your mind and loosen tensed-up muscles.

- Like the actors in certain old movies, splash some water on your face to relax tight facial muscles and refocus your thoughts.
- Wiggle your toes and fingers. This will stimulate circulation at your extremities, plus provide a physical outlet for the energy your system wants to expend.
- Take advantage of your body's readiness for action by exercising, washing the car, or getting some other necessary chore accomplished. When anxiety hits, sitting and stewing is the last thing you ought to do. So why not redirect yourself to a productive task that will not only alleviate stress now but also cross an item or two off this

Right:
Laughter really is the best medicine; don't be afraid to be silly!

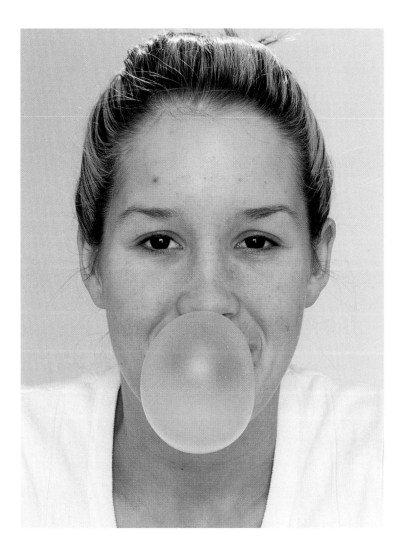

week's "to do" list? Also, if you choose to exercise, make your workout aerobic. Aerobic exercise causes hormones called endorphins to be released from the brain into your bloodstream. These hormones are known to have a mildly narcotic, calming effect that distance runners often refer to as "runner's high."

- Take a nice, hot bath with liberal quantities of your favorite aromatic bath salts. The warmth of the water will enhance blood flow, open your nasal passages, and relax your muscles, all of which are conducive to the immediate relief of stress. As for the scented bath salts, we must admit that the scientific community is divided about whether aromatherapy works exactly as advertised. But on the other hand, anything that makes you feel as though you are immersed in fragrant lavender or freshly cut cedar boughs can't be all bad, now, can it?

- Run to the store and get yourself some bubbles to blow. Here again, we can't offer any heavy-duty medical reason as to why blowing bubbles helps take the edge off of stress; we just know that it does. A little dose of silliness in any form, perhaps, is good medicine for stress relief.

Big Picture Suggestions

- Avoid unnecessary stress whenever possible. If, for example, you constantly argue with your younger sister because she dips into your cosmetics bag without asking, try buying some makeup for her. In a single bold stroke, you will have eliminated a major source of exasperation in your life, displayed your generosity and maturity, restored peace to the household, and perhaps even shamed the little witch into behaving better next time . . . all for the cost of a couple of lipsticks, some eyeliner, and a bottle of mascara. Be careful, however, that you don't sidestep life's necessary challenges in the name of stress avoidance. If you are struggling with math, for instance, you do yourself no favors by feigning a cold to miss a test in trig. That's stress deferral, not stress avoidance.

- Try to solve your problems, as opposed to dwelling on them. To pick up our previous example about the trig class, we'd suggest that you respond to your anxieties by taking practical measures to solve the problem that's behind them—in this case, your weak math skills and the fear of performing poorly. Possible remedies might include asking the teacher to work with you after hours, seeking the assistance of a tutor, or studying with other students who excel in the subject. How many people do you know who routinely spend hours on end fretting over their schoolwork, their jobs, or their relationships, yet next to no time at all on seriously addressing the underlying issues that vex them? We certainly know a few—and their problems just seem to get worse and worse!

Below:

A bit of stress now and then may be just what you need to get motivated for a big test or other challenge.

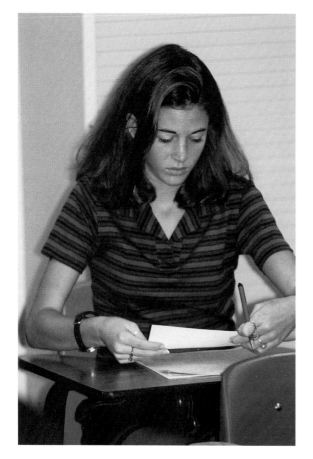

- To borrow from the title of a national bestseller, don't sweat the small stuff. Trust us, many of the concerns that seem monumental to you today will seem laughable in time. If you doubt it, just think back to the stuff you worried about back when you were 8 or 9.

- In similar fashion, try to get a solid understanding of what's really important in your life. Meditation and yoga are two popular ways to find balance in a hectic world. Once you know your priorities, it's easier to filter out the noise of day-to-day irritations and not allow them to deflect your attention from more meaningful matters.

- Under all circumstances, keep your sense of humor. It will not only help see you through the tough times in life, but also make the good times even better.

- When things get really bad and you feel out of control, seek the help of professionals and support groups. There is no disgrace in conceding that you need assistance—whether it comes in the form of an antianxiety drug prescribed by a physician, a group therapy session with others in the same circumstance, or the trusted advice of an analyst or counselor.

Keep It Cool, But Not Too Cool

As a general rule, you want to keep yourself away from stressful situations. But this doesn't mean that stress itself can't serve a useful purpose from time to time. Stress can be the wake-up call that informs you of the need to end a bad relationship or to mend a good one that's somehow gone sour. Stress can get you geared up for the challenge of a big job interview, a big test, a big game. Stress can even save your life by sharpening your senses while you drive on a busy highway. So keep it cool, but not too cool: An occasional dose of moderate stress is not only acceptable, but often beneficial.

LAST, BUT NOT LEAST: SLEEP

After you've taken pains to eat all the right foods, get some exercise, and skillfully manage the stress in your life, one item still remains on your "smart-living" checklist—SLEEP. Sweet, refreshing, rejuvenating sleep. On the surface, it may seem as though nothing much happens while you snooze, aside from the odd dream you recall the next morning. But this is misleading. Sleep is actually a very productive period for your entire body. Children, adolescents, and teens, for instance, do most of their growing while asleep; and bed rest is routinely recommended for the sick because that is when we heal fastest. At night, the body gets the opportunity to slow down, relax and most important, repair itself.

Not surprisingly, nighttime is the skin's best chance to undo all the damage we subject it to on a daily basis. The relief comes, in part, from what sleep denies us, such as exposure to UV radiation, smog, dirt, makeup, and stress. In addition, sleep gives our facial skin (and the muscles beneath it) a well-deserved respite from serving as the mirror of our thoughts and emotions. When we're awake, we create wrinkles without even knowing it, just by talking, smiling, frowning, and performing the wide range of movements that make our daytime faces so animated

PRODUCT SPOTLIGHT   Nighttime Skin Care

Sleep helps those who help themselves. While getting the right amount of shuteye is vital to your skin's well-being, it takes your active involvement to get a real beauty boost out of sleep. First, clean up your act. Some women make the mistake of going to sleep with their makeup on. This causes dry skin to become drier, and oily skin to become more oily. Once you've come clean, many dermatologists recommend overnight use of creams or lotions containing alpha-hydroxy acid (or AHA) to gently exfoliate the skin. By sloughing off the dead cells of the skin's top layer during the wee hours, you can put your freshest face forward the next day. Why at night? Because AHA unearths virgin layers of skin, which renders your face more sensitive to solar radiation. If you use these products in the daytime, you therefore increase the possibility of suffering a nasty burn. Besides, a pre-sleep application guarantees several hours of uninterrupted treatment.

Many AHA products, such as Basis All Night Face Cream and Nivea's Inner Beauty Nighttime Renewal Creme contain a built-in moisturizer. If you're using one that doesn't, yet still wish to moisturize, *be sure to apply the moisturizer on top of your AHA cream or lotion*. Otherwise, the AHA may never reach your skin.

Is your skin getting all the vitamins it needs in your daytime diet? If not, some scientists now believe that certain vitamins retain their skin-friendly properties when applied topically. The leading letter in this trend is antioxidant vitamin A. Vitamin A is thought to penetrate the skin to combat free radicals caused by exposure to environmental hazards like UV rays and pollution, which wreak havoc with the skin on a cellular level. Origins' vitamin-packed Night-A-Mins is an aromatherapeutic product designed to not only help you nod off via soothing neroli and valerian but also ward off those menacing free radicals. Dermatologica's Intensive Moisture Balance may also protect and defend your sleeping skin with antioxidants A, C, and E.

If you really want to go all out, you can also set yourself up with a slew of pampering facial moisturizers that positively love to work the late shift. A great place to start is the thin, delicate skin around your eyes, which absorbs daily abuse not only through the effects of squinting and blinking but also through the rubbing, tugging, and pulling required to apply and remove eye makeup. When choosing an overnight moisturizer, however, be careful to select one that's safe and gentle enough for use in this sensitive region. It should not irritate the eyelids or the tender skin surrounding the eyes, nor should it sting or burn if you accidentally get some in the eye itself. SkinMedica Rejuvenative Night Cream, Neutrogena Night Repair Cream, and Oil of Olay Night Cream will all give you the combination of effectiveness and gentleness you want.

The eyes aren't the only area of the face that can benefit from special bedside treatment. Since many of us sleep with our mouths open, lips can easily become dried out and chapped while we snooze. To smooth things over and seal in moisture, apply a thin coating of petroleum jelly as a protective measure. While you have the jar out, spread some over other dry, rough,

spots such as the palms of your hands and the soles of your feet, then pull on lightweight cotton gloves and socks to keep the sheets free of grease.

Of course, none of this over-the-counter TLC will amount to much if you can't fall asleep. Fortunately, aromatherapists have burned the midnight oil to determine which scents can help the sleep-deprived get their beauty rest. Vanilla, cedar wood, lavender, and chamomile, in particular, have been shown to produce relaxing effects, which may help ease you into sleep. Two to try: Bath & Body Works Tranquil Sleep Linen Spray, which offers tranquil aromas of vanilla, cedar wood, and clary sage; and Origins' Slumber Party Sensory Therapy Airspray, a fragrant and blissfully calming blend of star anise, tansy, bergamot, and honey myrtle. To use either, just spritz lightly onto sheets, set the alarm, and fill your mind with happy thoughts for the sweet dreams ahead.

and expressive. But when we sleep, this constant pulling, twisting, and stretching stops, thereby easing facial tension. It's like taking off a shirt you've worn all day and hanging it up: the wrinkles tend to fall out.

Antiwrinkling processes also take place during the slow wave portion of the sleep cycle, commonly known as "deep sleep." When we sleep our soundest, the body produces greater quantities of estrogen and progesterone—two hormones that help prevent the thinning of the skin that contributes to the development of wrinkles as we age. Over the years, too many lost hours of hormone-producing sleep may leave you with skin that's not only less youthful and vibrant but also more acne-prone than it would have been otherwise. Sun damage, too, is repaired during the hours we spend out of harm's way. Because a sleeping body isn't distracted by keeping up with daytime activities like walking and chewing gum, it can devote a much more generous percentage of its energy and resources to replacing scorched epidermal cells and mending broken-down collagen and elastin fibers. Way back at the beginning of this book, we mentioned that the skin possesses an almost miraculous capacity to bounce back from adversity. But to maximize these remarkable self-healing powers, you must afford your skin the luxury of some free time in the form of adequate sleep.

How Many Z's Do You Need Nightly?

Below:
Don't cheat yourself on sleep—it's essential for looking and feeling your best.

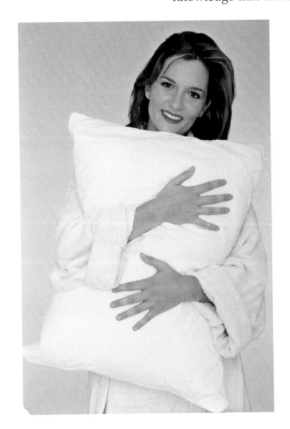

Everyone needs a different amount of sleep. Some of us can function quite well on as little as 6 hours of sleep per night, while others may require a full 8 hours or more. It's common knowledge that teens in general tend to be heavy sleepers—and with good reason! The rapid growth and maturation that occurs during this stage of life makes getting some extra Z's an absolute necessity, especially since our bodies typically stop growing sometime in early adulthood. As a result, the teen who shortchanges herself on sleep today creates a developmental deficit that cannot be made up later. Erratic sleep patterns also have consequences in the here and now, such as increased irritability, memory lapses, poor concentration, and a generally haggard appearance. Conversely, research shows that people who get their fair share of sleep are usually less prone to moodiness, more productive, and better able to absorb and retain information than those who do not.

If you wonder whether you're getting enough rest, a glance in the mirror will often answer the question for you. Gaunt, pale skin, bags or circles under the eyes, and a pasty, sallow complexion are all signs that you probably should have gotten to bed earlier—or stayed there longer. The best advice is to listen to your body, taking note of the circumstances that pertain when you feel well rested and refreshed on waking, as well as those that pertain when you get out of bed feeling groggy and lifeless. Be attentive in this process, and you will receive valuable clues regarding both your optimal bedtime and the number of sleep hours your body needs.

10 Tips for Better Sleep

Most of us have some trouble sleeping every now and again. Often we find it difficult to put the cares, concerns, and pressures of the recently completed day behind us, and so enter the bedroom in an agitated, wakeful state. While the following ten tips will not cure you of a serious or chronic sleep disorder—for that, you want a specialist—they can help you prepare your mind and body for a good night's rest. Follow them, and you will hopefully lay your head on the pillow tonight feeling receptive to sleep and freed, at least until morning, from the worries of the moment.

1. **Make your bedroom a pleasant place to be** (and sleep!). Decorate with your favorite photographs, choose soothing colors for the walls and accents, and add candles to your bedside. Flowers are also nice to notice and smell, so long as they aren't so fragrant as to be distracting.

2. **Follow the natural human sleep pattern** by going to bed early and rising early. Also, once you fall into a sleep groove that works for you, try to stick with it. Your nightly routine ought to help you gradually transition from the hustle and bustle of the day to the peace and tranquility of the sleep that awaits you.

3. **Unwind physically.** Progressively relax your body, gently tensing and then releasing each group of muscles. Yoga and meditation, in particular, are great for relaxation.

4. **Unwind mentally** by clearing your mind of all anxieties and worrying thoughts of the day.

5. Tell yourself during the day—and again at night—that you will **relax in mind and body,** drift off to sleep effortlessly, and doze straight through until the next morning.

6. **Repeat a soothing, reassuring statement** to yourself or listen to a tape recording of rhythmic, natural sounds (waves gently splashing on the beach, a spring breeze lightly rustling the leaves of a tree) when you first lie down. These are the "big girl" equivalents of the lullabies that probably helped you nod off as an infant.

7. **Try drinking hot milk and honey, or a malted milk drink,** as a comforting bedtime beverage.

8. **Don't read an exciting book or watch a suspenseful movie** just before going to bed. Even if the story isn't especially scary or tragic, simply getting mentally and/or emotionally involved in it can be enough to keep you awake well past bedtime.

9. **Avoid nicotine, caffeine, and other stimulants** for at least an hour prior to bedtime, and preferably longer. Many people, in fact, find that their sleep becomes disrupted or delayed if they have a second cup of coffee at lunchtime.

10. **Try not to worry if you don't fall asleep right away,** as this is a virtually foolproof way of ensuring continued wakefulness. Instead of fretting over the amount of sleep you're losing, console yourself with this fact: You will derive most of the benefits of real sleep through mere rest and relaxation. So lie still, close your eyes, put your mind at peace, and let your body relax.

END NOTES

1. In similar fashion, serious skin problems caused by dietary deficiencies are extremely infrequent nowadays. The classic example of such a disorder is scurvy, a skin disease that is brought about by lack of vitamin C and marked by bleeding gums; swollen, puffy skin; and a tendency to bruise easily. In the old days before refrigeration, sea-bound sailors—who often spent months on end away from land and thus had no access to fresh fruit—were especially prone to this dangerous ailment.

2. The National Cancer Institute estimates that reductions of 15% to 50% could be achieved in the incidence of certain cancers if Americans derived a greater percentage of their calories from vegetables and fruits than they currently do. These cancers include colon and rectal cancer, breast cancer, as well as prostate, endometrium, and gallbladder cancer.

3. It's important to note that all oils—even vegetable oils—are 100% fat and add around 135 calories per tablespoon to whatever dish you're preparing. That's why health experts try to steer people away from frying as a food preparation method. If you must fry, though, vegetable oils are the better choice because they are composed of monounsaturated fat rather than saturated fat.

4. Prescription supplements or over-the-counter supplements recommended by your doctor, of course, are an entirely different matter. These are often prescribed for people with severe digestive conditions or for chemotherapy patients who have trouble holding down regular food.

5. If this sounds familiar, it should! As you'll recall from Chapter Four, "That Four-Letter Word: Zit," vitamin A (in the form of tretinoin) is used as an active ingredient in acne-fighting drugs like Retin-A, as well as in other skin care medications.

6. The term B complex (abbreviated B_c) does not apply to an individual vitamin but to any chemical compound formed by the mixture of several B vitamins. We've listed niacin and folic acid as surrogate names for vitamin Bc, but many others, including thiamin and riboflavin, could have been listed as well.

7. Recent evidence suggests that folic acid, which is found naturally in citrus fruits and juices, may help prevent birth defects in the babies of mothers who consume at least 400 µg of it daily. Better still, consumption of folic acid—in combination with a healthy diet and sound prenatal care—can prevent up to 70% of the most dangerous kinds of birth defects: those of the brain and spine.

8. For a copy of the EAT Test, see pages 341-343 in Janis Jibrin's fine book, *The Unofficial Guide To Dieting Safely* (Macmillan, 1998).

9. This is the women's scale. For men, the standard is 106 pounds

at 5 feet in height, plus 6 additional pounds for every inch above 5 feet.

10. Dieticians and health writers often distinguish between "good" cholesterol and "bad" cholesterol. The good cholesterol is known by the acronym HDL (short for high-density lipoprotein); the bad, by the acronym LDL (or low-density lipoprotein). Elevated LDL levels are associated with cardiovascular disease because this type of cholesterol tends to form fatty deposits along artery walls, thus clogging the smooth flow of blood and stressing the heart. HDL cholesterol, by constrast, plays the role of a scavenger and actually removes these dangerous fats from your bloodstream. Regular exercise is one of the best ways to raise your HDL level, which in turn should serve to lower your LDL level.

11. For a much more complete discussion of this topic and aerobic exercise in general, readers are encouraged to consult the work of Dr. Kenneth Cooper, who has published a number of authoritative books and articles on the subject.

NOTES

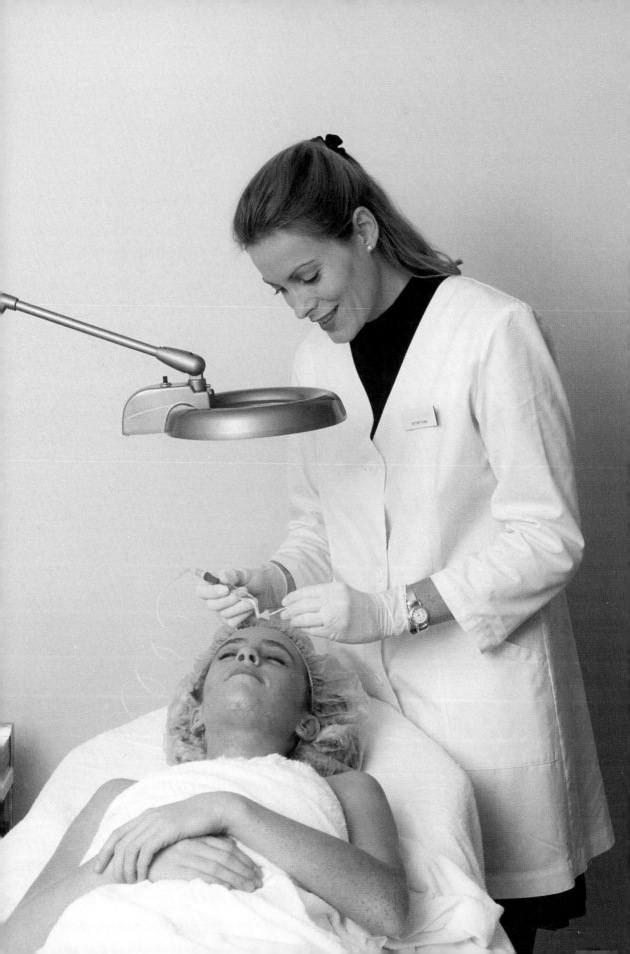

Finding Dr. Right: How To Choose Your Dermatologist

Dermatologists, as we noted way back in Chapter One, are doctors with specialized training about the skin. They learn to diagnose and treat diseases and conditions specific to the skin, such as eczema and psoriasis, as well as to detect broader illnesses whose symptoms result in changes and/or damage to the skin. Examples of the latter include the yellowing of the complexion that usually occurs when someone is suffering from hepatitis, or the "butterfly rash" that often emerges on the face of a lupus victim.[1]

THE DERMATOLOGIST'S TRAINING

An American dermatologist's schooling and training typically consist of:

- Four years of conventional undergraduate college study
- Four years of medical school (where he or she learns the same things your everyday doctor or family physician does)
- One to three years of on-the-job training in surgery, general medicine, or a mix of the two (this period, in combination with the next in our list, is referred to as a doctor's *internship* or *residency*)
- Three additional years of intense training and instruction exclusively in the skin (referred to as *residency specialty training*)

The final step for prospective dermatologists is to pass national board exams in their specialty. After that hurdle has been cleared, they are allowed to set up shop as Board Certified Dermatologists, which means they can start seeing, diagnosing, and treating patients on their own. You should always make sure that your doctor is not only certified, but has also maintained his or her certification over the years. The government, you see, requires practicing dermatologists—and other kinds of doctors, for that matter—to take "continuing medical education" courses to ensure that they stay up-to-date with the most recent advances in medical science.

WHAT THE DERMATOLOGIST TREATS

You'd figure, after this much instruction, that any old dermatologist would know just about everything there is to know about the skin and the problems that afflict it. But our bodies are so complex, and the pace of modern medical research is so fast, that no one individual can realistically master every aspect of the discipline. Nearly all dermatologists, however, are capable of diagnosing and treating the most common conditions encountered in day-to-day practice. These "normal" skin problems cover a wider range of ailments than you might initially imagine. A short list of them would include:

- Allergic contact dermatitis, or an inflammation of the skin sparked by direct physical exposure to certain plants (most often, poison ivy, poison oak, or poison sumac) or other substances to which an individual may be allergic (nickel, chrome, and the parabens contained in some cosmetics and salves are common offenders)

- Seborrheic dermatitis, the term used to describe rashes—often accompanied by yellowish scales—that crop up in oily regions of the skin like the eyebrows, ears, chest, central face, navel, and scalp
- Pigmentation problems—or abnormalities in pigmentation—such as moles, dark spots, light spots, birthmarks, and blotchy patches
- Acne in all its manifestations (whiteheads, blackheads, cysts, etc.)
- Sunburn, skin cancers, and sun damage in general
- Fungal (or yeast) infections of the skin, nails, and hair wherever they occur, though the most typical areas affected are in regions predisposed to chafing, such as the groin, the vagina, the cuticles, the nail folds, the corners of the mouth, inside the mouth, and under the breasts
- Warts, cold sores, and other skin conditions caused by viral invaders
- Impetigo, boils, and other skin conditions caused by bacterial invaders
- Hand, foot, and nail problems such as corns, bunions, ingrown toenails, calluses, and hangnails
- Hair problems like dandruff, hirsutism, and the various hair loss disorders we discussed in Chapter Five
- Chronic (or recurring) skin conditions such as psoriasis or eczema
- Traumatic injuries to the skin, including those brought about by insect bites, stings, burns, and frostbite

A good everyday dermatologist, then, can help you keep your skin free of trouble from the tips of your toenails to the top of your head. Ideally, though, your dermatologist will do more for you (and your skin!) than provide treatment when you have problems requiring medical attention. He or she can also serve as a valuable resource for skin-related advice of all kinds. Does your skin itch a lot? Perhaps it's too dry, and your doctor can figure out whether you ought to start using a moisturizer or simply need to avoid certain activities or products that tend to dehydrate the skin. Are you having trouble finding a shampoo that leaves your hair clean and manageable? Then ask your dermatologist for guidance. Unlike a hair stylist, he or she probably doesn't get a commission from you choosing one brand over another. Considering a tattoo? Well, your dermatologist cannot only give you pointers about what to look for in a parlor by way of sanitation and hygiene, but can also tell you what it will take to remove that tattoo should you later decide you don't like it.

Ultimately, this type of preventive care and consultation can be every bit as beneficial to the health of your skin as the direct medical treatment you'll occasionally receive from your dermatologist. Perhaps even more so. But it takes time and familiarity for a doctor to be able to serve you in this manner. Over the course of many years, dermatologists pick up valuable nuggets of information about their patients, not all of which are typically found in a file folder. A sharp doctor who has learned through casual conversation that you love water sports, for instance, will keep an eagle eye out for early signs of photo-aging and skin cancer, even if you don't have any suspicious looking moles or pigmentation problems right now. In addition, the diagnosis and treatment of many skin problems—such as identifying the source of an allergic reaction or finding the correct medication to deal with a specific strain of problem acne—can often require months of cooperative effort by both doctor and patient.

As a result, it really pays to find a dermatologist you like and trust, then stick with him or her so that you can derive the full benefits of a solid, long-term doctor-patient relationship. For all of these reasons, you want to be selective and find just the right doctor for you. We suggest a thorough, three-step approach.

STEP ONE: FINDING A MATCH

Once certified, some dermatologists choose to establish their own place of business and open a clinic; others take a partner or team up with peers in other specialties to create small medical centers; and still others prefer to work within the framework of a larger institution such as a hospital or research facility. Of course, it doesn't much matter where your doctor's office is located or whether it is connected with a hospital or not. The important issues are to know that the dermatologist is completely qualified, has maintained credentials through ongoing certification, and operates his or her practice to high standards. You can get this information by checking with the appropriate state agencies and professional associations[2] to learn if the doctor has ever been reprimanded or sanctioned; by soliciting recommendations from family members, friends and acquaintances; and by talking directly to the dermatologist in question before you patronize the practice.

STEP TWO: ARE YOU COMPATIBLE?

This idea may seem somewhat bold, but (a) we're bold anyhow, right?; (b) it's a perfectly logical thing to do; and (c) a good doctor won't mind a bit. In fact, the better the doctor, the greater the likelihood that he or she will want to discuss his or her qualifications and practice. What's more, a thorough first interview gives you the chance to find out how much the dermatologist knows about the condition or illness that sent you to his or her door in the first place. Has the doctor treated this problem before? If so, how many times? Is it an area of special expertise? If so, what has the success rate been? And how does that success rate compare to national averages? These are all very relevant questions, and you owe it to yourself to receive clear, meaningful answers to them. Frankly, a good doctor wouldn't handle a rare disorder with which he or she was relatively unacquainted. Instead, he or she would refer the patient to a colleague with more hands-on experience, and expect colleagues to return the favor in cases where the reverse applied.

STEP THREE: TYING THE KNOT

For purposes of discussion, though, let's assume you've found a doctor who has come to you with an impeccable record, glowing referrals, and strong technical expertise, particularly in the areas that concern you most. Are you finished in your search? Close, but not quite. You need to go one step farther and find someone you like, trust, and respect as a person, and who will extend those same attitudes to you. That's because your relationship with any doctor—and especially your dermatologist—involves the sharing of details about your body, health, and lifestyle that are sometimes quite personal. Perhaps you (no, scratch that, someone you know) fears that she may be suffering from a sexually transmitted disease, because of the cold sores on her lips; or on a less dramatic level, notices that her feet have recently begun to stink to high heaven every time she slips off her shoes. In either case, your friend will be far more likely to overcome her self-consciousness and seek care right away if she's comfortable with her care giver. On the other hand, even an exceptionally talented dermatologist can't help her a jot if she finds herself unable, for whatever reason, to speak fully and candidly under all circumstances. It's therefore extremely important to choose a doctor who puts you at ease, displays a genuine concern for your well-being, listens attentively, and encourages an open, two-way exchange of information on all matters relating to the health and wellness of your skin.

Now that you know what to look for, get out there and find the perfect professional partner to help you keep your skin healthy and attractive. If you choose wisely, you will have taken an essential step toward maintaining your youthful complexion for a lifetime.

WHAT YOUR DERMATOLOGIST NEEDS TO KNOW ABOUT YOU

The doctor-patient relationship is based on trust and protected by confidentiality. Thus you, as a patient, have certain obligations that must be fulfilled if you expect your dermatologist to provide the best care possible. In particular, a doctor needs a lot of information to do his or her job well. To care for you effectively and safely, he or she must know about:

- Your complete medical history
- Any health problems that run in your family
- Any chronic illnesses you suffer from (whether they affect the skin or not)
- Any drugs you're taking that have been prescribed by other doctors
- Your lifestyle in a general sense, but especially those aspects of it that may affect skin health (Do you smoke? Drink alcohol? Sunbathe? Lose sleep due to long work hours? Etc.)

END NOTES

1. Lupus is a potentially deadly autoimmune disorder that typically afflicts young women in their late 20s and early 30s. The rash gets its name because it originates near the bridge of the nose, then spreads out (like butterfly wings) along both cheekbones, just under the eye sockets.

2. One excellent source of information is the American Academy of Dermatology. You can contact them by mail at PO Box 4014, 930 N. Meacham Road, Schaumburg, IL 60168-4014; or via the Internet at http://www.aad.com. To reach the organization by phone, call 847-330-0230; by fax, 847-330-0050.

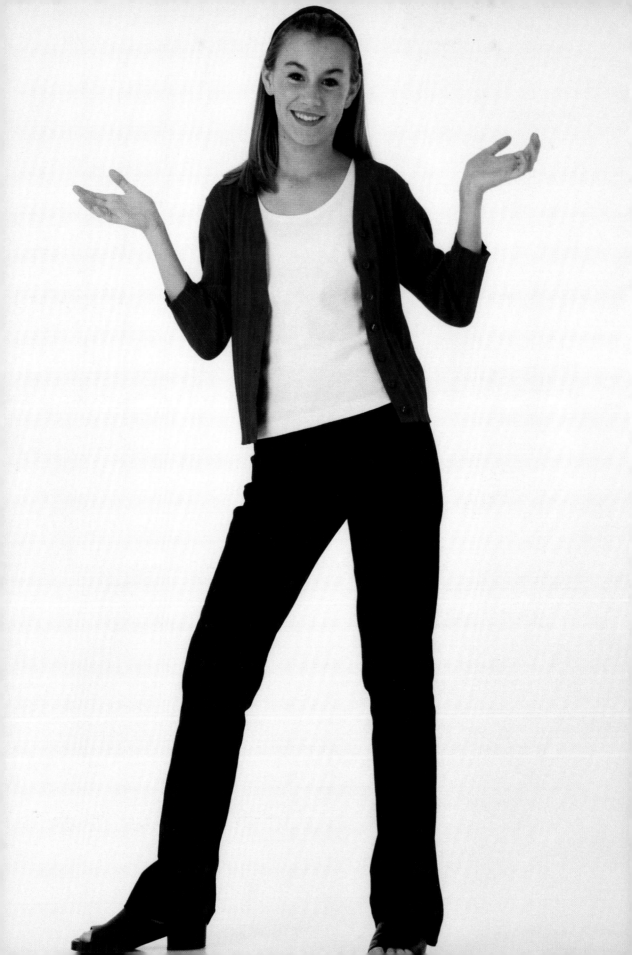

The Last Word:
A Summary of Key Points

Popular culture today sends mixed messages to young women on the subject of beauty. On the one hand, there is the indirect—but very real—pressure to be as drop-dead gorgeous as the supermodels and actresses whose images pervade our lives through magazine ads, billboards, TV shows, movies, and now even via our home computers. Frankly, this media-driven beauty blitz sets a standard that no woman can hope to attain. After all, even the most striking professional models, who start out with a high degree of natural beauty and spend hours every day focusing exclusively on their looks, don't pop out of bed at 6 AM ready to face the camera. They, too, must weather bad hair days, cope with skin problems, watch their weight, and deal with insecurities about their appearance far more often than the smiling, self-assured images on the magazine covers suggest. In fact, if a model strolled past you in a busy mall, wearing her ordinary clothes and light makeup, our guess is that you wouldn't find it easy to distinguish her from dozens of other attractive women who just happened to be shopping at the same time. Hey, ideals are great. They give us something to shoot for. But when you combine an unrealistic standard of feminine beauty with a culture that puts a premium on the appearance of its women, the results can be damaging and, in some cases, devastating. Consequently, many teenage women feel that they can never look quite good enough, and thus suffer from unwarranted feelings of inadequacy and low esteem.

On the other hand, young women who are fortunate enough to be blessed with good looks may face the equally pervasive—and much more direct—pressure of old-fashioned human envy. It is a sad fact of life that people will both admire and despise you for your strengths, no matter what form they take. For every beautiful woman who is unfairly labeled as a "ditz" or "dumb blonde," there is an athletic young man somewhere being called a "stupid jock" and a future molecular biologist whose classmates dismiss her as a "geek." In the end, it seems, you just can't win. You are encouraged by the culture around you to be as physically attractive as a *Glamour* covergirl, but not so attractive as to arouse the envy of your peers. Further, you are expected to attend to your appearance and attire to a degree that no man would ever dream of, yet still find time to excel in school, stay fit, hold down a part-time job, and be helpful around the house. What a load! Adults who say that teen life is a breeze have forgotten what it's like to be a teen.

While we can't tell you how to juggle all the conflicting pressures and demands in your life (we're juggling our own, and balls keep hitting the ground!), we can offer some thoughts on what we feel is a sensible approach to beauty. Please understand that these are simply our opinions, not matters of scientific fact. You are free to accept or reject them as you see fit. But we do believe they are valuable—in some ways every bit as valuable as the practical advice we've offered in this book—because they are intended to help you view and use beauty as a means of cultivating that most critical of all internal resources, self esteem.

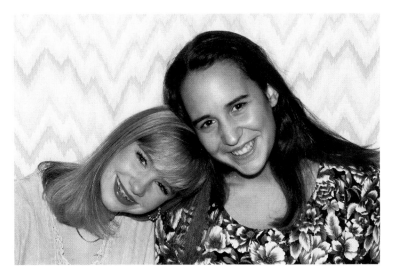

Left:
Accentuate the positive and celebrate your own unique beauty!

For us, a sensible approach to beauty means…

• **Appreciating and accentuating the unique attributes that make each of us beautiful,** though in different ways. Is Lauren Hutton's gap-toothed grin an aesthetic flaw that ought to be corrected? Or a signature feature that gives us a brief and tantalizing glimpse of the woman within? Well, the camera, along with 99% of America, seems to have voted in favor of the latter. And we do, too. In fact, we say hooray for Lauren Hutton and all other women, famous or not, who possess the perspective, self-confidence, and good sense to realize that beauty doesn't spring from some static ideal but from the very real physical, mental, and emotional differences that set us apart from every other human being on the planet. So when you look in the mirror, you shouldn't constantly be searching for flaws. Instead, try looking for those defining characteristics, physical and otherwise, that make you special. Then play them up to the hilt!

• **Setting priorities and establishing goals:** You'll spend at least some portion of every living day taking care of your skin, hair, and nails, so it's worthwhile to ask yourself how highly you value your appearance and what you hope to achieve from your daily regimen. If your goal is to be a highly paid runway model some day, beauty will be a top priority and other facets of your life will have to take a back seat or be shelved altogether. If your goal is the more modest (and common) one of maintaining healthy skin and presenting a reasonably well-groomed appearance, beauty will probably rank as a relatively low priority, a task you try to dispense with as quickly and efficiently as possible. Either end of the spectrum is fine, as is anything in between. The important point is to have a purpose, be it great or small, when you walk into the bathroom every morning and night.

• **Budgeting your time:** Once you know your goals, this part becomes fairly easy—or, at worst, resolves itself through daily practice. The difficult thing is sticking to your plan and actually using the time you've mentally set aside for skin care and beauty. To protect it, always remember that this is *your private time*, that tiny fraction of each day during which you attend to your own needs and put yourself first. Even if you have only 20 minutes to wash your face, brush your hair, and apply makeup in the morning, be sure to block out all distractions and use every single second for the purpose at hand. Trust us, the demands of the real world will be there, waiting, the moment you are finished.

• **Working from a health-first perspective:** As you've seen countless times in the preceding pages, beautifying your skin begins with caring for it properly and protecting it from harm. Everything else is window dressing, by comparison—important, to be sure, but *not crucial*. In fact, the biggest bonus of having healthy skin, hair, and nails is that they don't require a lot of cosmetic doctoring to be made attractive. This not only saves you time and money, but also allows you to concentrate on improving your appearance, not repairing it. Finally, recall that the health of your skin can be affected for the better as much (and probably more) by what you avoid as by what you actively do. The best example: sun protection. Every hour that you spend away from—or heavily protected against—UV exposure today will save you countless hours in skin care down the line.

• **Understanding the true rewards of beauty and the reasons it's worth pursuing:** For Tyra Banks, beauty pays the rent—and then some! For the rest of us, the payoff is less tangible, but no less rewarding if we maintain our sense of perspective. Ideally, beauty should be an outward expression of a woman's inner sense of self-worth, a means of visibly demonstrating—to herself, perhaps, as much as to anyone else—that she not only cares deeply about her health and appearance, but also makes a conscious effort to foster both. Some might argue that it is selfish and small-minded to cultivate physical beauty. But these people miss the point: The pursuit of beauty is selfish only when it becomes a preoccupation; that is, when other important aspects of life (such as intellectual development or maintaining relationships) are sacrificed at its expense. For the vast majority of women who strive to look their best every day, this simply isn't the case. They pursue beauty not to the exclusion of other interests and obligations, but in addition to them. When all is said and done, such women take pride in their looks because they take pride in themselves as complete, well-rounded human beings. You should, too.

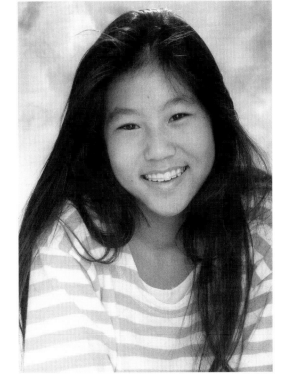

Above:
She's got the glow . . .

KEEPING THE GLOW: 13 EASY STEPS!

To close this book, we have summarized below thirteen of the key points made in the text. We hope you'll refer to this summary from time to time in the future as a periodic reminder of what you must do to keep the glow of beautiful, youthful-looking skin for a lifetime. The last page in this chapter has been purposely left blank so that you can jot down any ideas or tips you come across that are especially relevant to your personal skin care and beauty regimen but that haven't been included in our more general list.

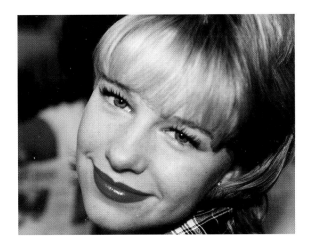

Above:
. . . She does too—and so can you!

1. **Don't smoke.** Nicotine is one of the most addictive and physically damaging drugs known to man, and ought to

be shunned by anyone who cares about their health and appearance. If you haven't started smoking, DON'T. If you have, quit now before years of addiction rob you of your capacity to drop this deadly habit. For similar reasons, say no to recreational drugs and avoid abuse of both alcohol and prescription medications. You will live a longer and happier life for having done so, and the results of your good judgment will be reflected in the mirror each and every morning.

2. **Avoid UV exposure** whenever you can, and protect yourself from the sun with appropriate clothing and SPF 30 or higher sunblock when you can't. This is the single best thing you can do for the long-term health of your skin. Period.

3. **Stay physically fit** with a minimum of 20 to 30 minutes of aerobic exercise at least three times a week.

4. **Eat a healthy, balanced diet** that's high in carbohydrates, protein, nutrients, and fiber but low in saturated fats and empty calories. Drink plenty of water, too: At a minimum, you need at least eight 8-ounce servings daily to satisfy your body's needs.

5. **Get your beauty rest.**

6. **Find a qualified dermatologist** to treat your skin problems and help you maintain skin health.

7. **Wash your face twice a day**—three times tops—with a cleanser suitable to your skin type.

8. **Always exercise a light, gentle touch when washing** your face and hair.

9. **Never try to handle problem acne on your own**, and never, ever pop a zit. Even relatively mild cases of acne can cause permanent scarring if mishandled. A qualified dermatologist can help you avoid the worst mistakes and put you on the path to proper treatment.

10. **Wash your hair regularly** with a shampoo that suits your hair type, but avoid overwashing like the plague.

11. **Keep your nails moisturized**, and give them an occasional respite from all nail care products.

12. **Use hypoallergenic cosmetics** that suit your skin type, and always wash them off completely before you go to

bed. If you are prone to breakouts, look for oil-free formulations that are both non-acnegenic and non-comedogenic.

13. **Continue to learn everything you can about your skin** and how to care for it. The fact that you've read this book is a terrific first step, but there are many other excellent sources of information out there, and new skin care breakthroughs are taking place with lightning speed. To keep current, make regular visits to your local library, explore the Internet, and read the skin care and beauty articles in your favorite women's magazines. All are chock full of useful information and helpful tips.

NOTES

Index